ANEMIA
PATIENT ADVOCATE

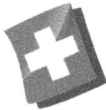

Health Scouter
WWW.HEALTHSCOUTER.COM

HealthScouter.com - Equity Press
5055 Canyon Crest Drive
Riverside, California 92507

www.healthscouter.com

Purchasing this book entitles you to free updates at www.healthscouter.com/Anemia

Edited By: Shana McKibbin

Includes Anemia from Wikipedia http://en.wikipedia.org/wiki/Anemia

HealthScouter Anemia: Symptoms of Anemia and Signs of Anemia: Anemia Patient Advocate (HealthScouter Anemia)

ISBN 978-1-60332-093-1

Important

NEVER DISREGARD PROFESSIONAL MEDICAL ADVICE, OR DELAY SEEKING IT, BECAUSE OF SOMETHING YOU HAVE READ IN THIS BOOK. ALWAYS SEEK PROFESSIONAL MEDICAL ADVICE BEFORE ACTING UPON INFORMATION READ IN THIS BOOK.

HealthScouter and Equity Press do not provide medical advice. The contents of this book are for informational purposes only and are not intended to substitute for professional medical advice, diagnosis or treatment. Always seek advice from a qualified physician or health care professional about any medical concern, and do not disregard professional medical advice because of anything you may read in this book or on a HealthScouter Web site. The views of individuals quoted in this book are not necessarily those of HealthScouter or Equity Press.

While this book is intended to be a medium for the exchange of information and ideas, it is not meant in any way to be a substitute for sound medical advice; neither should it be viewed as a trusted source of such advice. The views expressed in these messages are not those of any qualified medical association, and the publisher is not responsible for the validity of the information communicated herein or for consequences that may arise from acting upon this information. The publisher is not responsible for any content found in the book that may be deemed offensive, inappropriate, inaccurate or medically unsound. The information you find here is only for the purpose of discussion and should not be the basis for any medical decision. The content is not intended to be a substitute for professional medical advice, diagnosis or treatment.

The information presented is not to be considered complete, nor does it contain all medical resource information that may be relevant, and therefore it is not intended to be a substitute for seeking medical treatment and/or appropriate care.

By reading this book and parts of the Web site, you agree under all circumstances to hold harmless, and to refrain from seeking remedy from, the owners of this book. The publisher shall disclaim all liability to you for damages, costs or expenses, including legal and medical fees, related to your reliance on anything derived from this book or Web site or its contents. Furthermore, Equity Press assumes no liability for any and all claims arising out of the said use, regardless of the cause, effects, or fault.

Equity Press and HealthScouter do not endorse any company or product, and listing on the HealthScouter Web site is not linked to corporate sponsorship. We do not make a claim to being comprehensive or up to date. If you would like to recommend information to include in this book, please contact us – we would be very happy to hear from you.

Purchasing this book entitles you to free updates as they are available. Please register your book at www.healthscouter.com

TABLE OF CONTENTS

INTRODUCTION AND MOTIVATION

Dear Reader,

I like to think of myself as a polite, well-reasoned person. I rarely speak out or complain. When a waitress spills something on me, or if my meal is cold—or if I'm overcharged—I generally try to be as polite as possible. I don't like to make very many waves. I often secretly hope that the manager will hear about my predicament and come out and offer me a free meal, or something similar. I generally hope that my polite and respectful demeanor pays off. And it does happen from time to time. You know, I think many people are brought up to believe that this is just good manners. It's how you're supposed to behave. And if you knew me personally, I think you'd agree that I'm generally pretty reserved. Of course my wife may raise an objection or two (!), but I really believe that it's important to treat others as you would like to be treated. We're talking about the golden rule here—it works well and it applies to almost every life circumstance.

But I have to admit that when it comes to my health, or the health of someone I care about—all bets are off. I want to know what's going on—when, why, where, and how. And I make these feelings known. I tend to get downright assertive. It's just something I feel very strongly about. And I feel that when you are in a hospital, or if you're brushing up against the healthcare system, that you should feel the same way. It's unfamiliar turf, and the professionals who work in this system often take advantage of their positions. They may use some jargon to hide the whole truth— or they may say something without checking to make sure you understand completely. They may present the options that are best for them, perhaps the most profitable or convenient. Now I'm not saying this goes on everywhere. There are many professionals in the business of health who go out of their way to make sure you have the best care. And I'm not suggesting that you should become a bully, or purposefully annoying—absolutely not. But I am suggesting that I think it's OK for you to step outside of your typical comfort zone, and put on your patient advocate hat. Because you, the patient or patient advocate, care the most about your care—not the medical system or healthcare providers.

HealthScouter was created to help patients become better advocates for their own medical care. Because when it comes to your healthcare, the stakes are high. There are none higher. And healthcare is one area where consumers (us, the sick people) are notoriously unaware of their options. And that's why I'm publishing these books. To help you understand your options, and to help you get the best care possible. I want to help you become a better advocate for yourself and for your loved ones.

It's my sincere hope that you can take this book with you to the hospital, to be read in the waiting room or by the bedside—and when you see a relevant patient comment you can use this book to ask questions of your health care providers. My advice: Ask lots of questions! Providers are busy people who generally go about their business with little questioning, delivering care as they see fit—making quick decisions—and again, nobody is going to care as much about your health as you. So now, more than ever, you need tools at your disposal to get the best care possible. One of the tools at your disposal is this HealthScouter book and the material within. You need to be armed with questions, and you need to ask questions all of the time. And so the difficult part is now to understand the right questions to ask.

That brings me to an explanation of how these books are structured. HealthScouter books include a number of what we call patient comments. These patient comments are summaries of what people have experienced. They're first hand accounts of what you may expect. These experiences effectively help you "catch up," and understand what outcomes are possible. They expose you to the treatments are available, and provide insight as to potential outcomes. They help you understand what other people are doing. So if you find yourself stuck feeling like you're receiving substandard medical care—or if you need a push to broach the subject, you can take this book to your provider and say, "Hey, I read here that another patient had this treatment—is that an option for me? If not, Why?" I believe that other peoples' experience is the most valuable way for you to formulate and build a list of good questions for your healthcare providers.

That notion is at the core of the HealthScouter philosophy.

So HealthScouter, by providing patient comments about a particular medical condition, will help expose you to what other people have experienced about a particular medical problem. If you know what other people have experienced, you can better understand what your options are. You'll be better informed and you'll have some questions to ask—it'll be like you've had access to dozens of other people who have gone through the same thing you're going through. And so armed, maybe you'll be able to move through your condition and get back on the road to health, and maybe you'll be able to do this with more grace than I have. And that is my sincere wish.

It's also my wish that perhaps when a doctor or nurse sees this little blue book, that they'll think twice about the care they're about to provide—knowing that the owner is a little bit better prepared, a little bit better armed—and yes, maybe even downright assertive.

I hope this book helps.

Yours truly,

Jim Stewart

San Diego, California

HOW TO USE THIS BOOK

The purpose of HealthScouter is to help you understand your medical condition as quickly and easily as possible. We believe this can best be accomplished by reading about other people and their experiences negotiating their health and care. We try to leave out complicated medical jargon. And we've spent a considerable amount of time structuring this book so that it's easy to use. It's important to know that this is not the sort of book you read from beginning to end. Of course you may do so, but this book is more meaningful if you flip through quickly and scan for applicable material. Again, it's all about the patient commentary: The darkly shaded comments ▪ indicate one patient initiating a new discussion, and the light or clear comments ▭ are other comments associated with that same condition. So you should begin by looking for information from other patients who are experiencing the same aspect of the same medical condition that you studying. You can do this quickly by scanning through the book, focusing on the dark shaded comment boxes. By scanning the patient comments you'll find information about various aspects of a condition, all grouped together, in an easy-to-read format. In this way you can immediately begin reading about other patients and their experiences with your particular medical condition – and you can benefit immediately from their experiences.

INTRODUCTION TO ANEMIA

Anemia is a decrease in normal number of red blood cells (RBCs) or less than the normal quantity of hemoglobin in the blood.[1][2] However, it can include decreased oxygen-binding ability of each hemoglobin molecule due to deformity or lack in numerical development as in some other types of hemoglobin deficiency.

Since hemoglobin (found inside RBCs) normally carries oxygen from the lungs to the tissues, anemia leads to hypoxia (lack of oxygen) in organs. Since all human cells depend on oxygen for survival, varying degrees of anemia can have a wide range of clinical consequences.

The three main classes of anemia include excessive blood loss (acutely such as a hemorrhage or chronically through low-volume loss), excessive blood cell destruction (hemolysis) or deficient red blood cell production (ineffective hematopoiesis).

Anemia is the most common disorder of the blood. There are several kinds of anemia, produced by a variety of underlying causes. Anemia can be classified in a variety of ways, based on the morphology of RBCs, underlying etiologic mechanisms, and discernible clinical spectra, to mention a few.

There are two major approaches: the "kinetic" approach which involves evaluating production, destruction and loss[3], and the "morphologic" approach which groups anemia by red blood cell size. The morphologic approach uses a quickly available and cheap lab test as its starting point (the MCV). On the other hand, focusing early on the question of production may allow the clinician more rapidly to expose cases where multiple causes of anemia coexist.

Definition

The general definition of anemia is decrease in normal number of red blood cells (RBCs) or less than the normal quantity of hemoglobin in the blood.[1][2] More specifically, it is the concentration of hemoglobin, red blood cell volume, or red blood cell number.[4]

Sometimes, decreased blood volume (hypovolemia) is also included in anemia definition,[2] which, however, in case of hypovolemia caused by bleeding, indirectly causes decreased hemoglobin concentration because of shift of interstitial fluid to plasma in autoreperfusion. Still, other causes of hypovolemia, such as dehydration or vomiting, which not cause loss of red blood cells or hemoglobin, actually increase blood hemoglobin concentration, which is contrary to the general definition of anemia.

Anemia is generally strictly distinguished from hypoxemia, defined as decreased partial pressure of oxygen in blood,[5][6][7][8] although both conditions are causes of hypoxia.

Signs and Symptoms

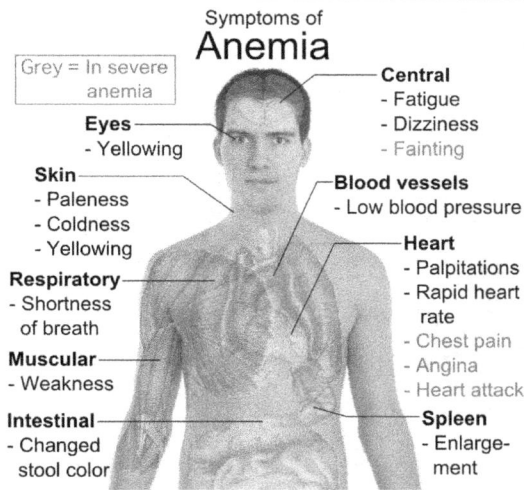

Symptoms of
Anemia

Grey = In severe anemia

Central
- Fatigue
- Dizziness
- Fainting

Eyes
- Yellowing

Skin
- Paleness
- Coldness
- Yellowing

Blood vessels
- Low blood pressure

Respiratory
- Shortness of breath

Heart
- Palpitations
- Rapid heart rate
- Chest pain
- Angina
- Heart attack

Muscular
- Weakness

Intestinal
- Changed stool color

Spleen
- Enlargement

Main symptoms that may appear in anemia.[9]

Anemia goes undetected in many people, and symptoms can be small and vague. The signs and symptoms can be related to the anemia itself, or the underlying cause.

Most commonly, people with anemia report non-specific symptoms of a feeling of weakness, or fatigue, general malaise and sometimes poor concentration. They may also report shortness of breath, dyspnea, on exertion. In very severe anemia, the body may compensate for the lack of oxygen carrying capability of the blood by increasing cardiac output. The patient may have symptoms related to this, such as palpitations, angina (if preexisting heart disease is present), intermittent claudication of the legs, and symptoms of heart failure.

On examination, the signs exhibited may include pallor (pale skin, mucosal linings and nail beds) but this is not a reliable sign. There may be signs of specific causes of anemia, e.g. koilonychia (in iron deficiency), jaundice (when anemia results from abnormal break down of red blood cells - in haemolytic anemia), bone deformities (found in thalassaemia major) or leg ulcers (seen in sickle cell disease).

In severe anemia, there may be signs of a hyperdynamic circulation: a fast heart rate (tachycardia), flow murmurs, and cardiac enlargement. There may be signs of heart failure.

Pica, the consumption of non-food based items such as dirt, paper, wax, grass, ice, and hair, may be a symptom of iron deficiency, although it occurs often in those who have normal levels of hemoglobin.

Chronic anemia may result in behavioral disturbances in children as a direct result of impaired neurological development in infants, and reduced scholastic performance in children of school age.

Restless legs syndrome is more common in those with iron deficiency anemia.

I am concerned about my daughter. She had blood tests done and they came back showing she is slightly anemic she is 15 and they are at 11.1, it also showed she has inflammation her levels for that were 29 and are supposed to be below 20. So they had her go back for a Ferritin level test, which came back normal. So they said she doesn't have iron deficiency anemia. About 1½ years ago she was diagnosed anemic and she was on an iron supplement for about nine months (doubling the dose halfway through) and only managed to get it up to 12.1. She is having bowel problems (Irritable Bowel symptoms).
So they had stool samples checked, we are still waiting on the fecal blood cultures but the other

tests are normal. She has horrible leg and joint pains a lot too but she has seen a rheumatologist before and they said it's not arthritis. Has anyone any ideas as to what this could be?

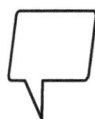

Has she had her B-12 and folate levels checked? This too can cause anemia unrelated to iron. Symptoms can also be body aches and pains. Reasons can be autoimmune related, did the rheumatologist check her for other things? Has she seen a gastroenterologist yet?

I was diagnosed with iron deficiency anemia about three months ago (I believe my hemo was 11 and my iron was 8 but I may have that backwards). I was put on two supplements daily. I have no other known health issues. I went to doctor because I was experiencing burning sensations on my skin (mostly back), itching, fatigue, acid reflux and nervousness/anxiety. Oh, and significant hair loss at hairline and sides. Within two weeks of treatment, most symptoms were completely gone, and hair is slowly coming in again.

My doctor went on maternity leave and the primary doctor said by phone that my new tests show iron and hemoglobin "coming up very nicely." He did not offer levels, but he did say I had to have a colonoscopy. (The fecal occult test came back negative). I am very upset about the prospect of undetected colon cancer to the point of being able to think about nothing else. I do not have ANY symptoms or risk factors or family history, other than perhaps eating too much dairy.

My youngest is three, but I only went off the prenatal vitamins a year and a half ago. Symptoms started in November.

Also, I get heavy periods, although not so heavy as to ever cause me to seek medical attention.

Has anyone else had numbers this low from diet and pregnancy/childbirth alone, or is it always an underlying disease or disorder?

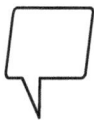

The colonoscopy does seem in order for the iron deficiency anemia to rule out any internal bleeding which is not necessarily a sign or symptom of cancer. You may also be scheduled for an upper endoscopy to check the stomach which can't be seen by the colonoscopy. In August 2008, I was diagnosed with IDA and even though my fecal occult test was negative for blood, I had to have *a colonoscopy even though I had had one in December 2006. The colonoscopy was negative. Since I had an upper endoscopy in March 2008, the gastroenterologist didn't feel it was necessary to repeat but instead did a capsule endoscopy to check the small intestine which isn't seen in either of the other scopes.*

Have you ever gotten a copy of the actual blood test? Are you being seen by a specialist or only a primary care provider? You have the right to request copies of any medical tests as well as any letters written by your specialist to your primary care provider. Please get copies and then post the results here and hopefully some of the "experts" will be able to help you understand.

I'm certainly not an expert since I'm still new to it all and trying to understand it all myself but from what I have read here, your heavy periods might be the culprit. I'm post-menopausal so that wasn't/ isn't my culprit. I do have acid reflux and take Nexium and that may be the cause. Seeing your gynecologist sounds like a good plan too.

Diagnosis

Generally, clinicians request complete blood counts in the first batch of blood tests in the diagnosis of an anemia. Apart from reporting the number of red blood cells and the hemoglobin level, the automatic counters also measure the size of the red blood cells by flow cytometry, which is an important tool in distinguishing between the causes of anemia. Examination of a stained blood smear using a microscope can also be helpful, and is sometimes a necessity in regions of the world where automated analysis is less accessible.

In modern counters, four parameters (RBC count, hemoglobin concentration, MCV and RDW) are measured, allowing others (hematocrit, MCH and MCHC) to be calculated, and compared to values adjusted for age and sex. Some counters estimate hematocrit from direct measurements.

WHO's Hemoglobin thresholds used to define anemia[10] (1 g/dL = 0.6206 mmol/L)		
Age or gender group	Hb threshold (g/dl)	Hb threshold (mmol/l)
Children (0.5–5.0 yrs)	11,0	6,8
Children (5–12 yrs)	11,5	7,1
Children (12-15 yrs)	12,0	7,4

Women, non-pregnant (>15yrs)	12,0	7,4
Women, pregnant	11,0	6,8
Men (>15yrs)	13,0	8,1

Reticulocyte counts, and the "kinetic" approach to anemia, have become more common than in the past in the large medical centers of the United States and some other wealthy nations, in part because some automatic counters now have the capacity to include reticulocyte counts. A reticulocyte count is a quantitative measure of the bone marrow's production of new red blood cells. The reticulocyte production index is a calculation of the ratio between the level of anemia and the extent to which the reticulocyte count has risen in response. If the degree of anemia is significant, even a "normal" reticulocyte count actually may reflect an inadequate response.

If an automated count is not available, a reticulocyte count can be done manually following special staining of the blood film. In manual examination, activity of the bone marrow can also be gauged qualitatively by subtle changes in the numbers and the morphology of young RBCs by examination under a microscope. Newly formed RBCs are usually slightly larger than older RBCs and show polychromasia. Even where the source of blood loss is obvious, evaluation of erythropoiesis can help assess whether the bone marrow will be able to compensate for the loss, and at what rate.

When the cause is not obvious, clinicians use other tests: ESR, ferritin, serum iron, transferrin, RBC folate level, serum vitamin B-12, hemoglobin electrophoresis, and renal function tests (e.g. serum creatinine).

When the diagnosis remains difficult, a bone marrow examination allows direct examination of the precursors to red cells.

I was diagnosed with Iron Deficiency Anemia in March 2008 and started 324mg iron supplements twice a day. I am ok with the side effects and all but am extremely confused as to why my levels have continued to drop in the last couple of months. My doctor says to continue the sup and come back in three months for re-check. Shouldn't my levels be rising or at least staying the same?

I have always had extremely heavy periods but since the birth of my twins in 2005 they last seven days and continuous bleeding. This is obviously the reason for the anemia but shouldn't

*the supplement be helping? Everything was ok
and normal in July of 2007 and then I went
downhill from there.*

*April 2008
Iron 91
TIBC 278
- FE SAT 33
Ferritin 18*

*June 2008
Iron 41
TIBC 262
% FE SAT 16
Ferritin 15*

*So what am I missing? I am worried about what
the levels will be the next time I go in. Is this
normal and does it take a while or what?*

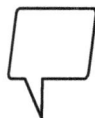

*If you are truly have very heavy periods (and it
sounds as if you are) the iron supplements really
won't be enough to combat the extensive blood
loss every month. In some people, they can stave
off the anemia, but your bleeding is probably too
heavy for that. I'm sure your pregnancy drained
you of any stores you had also.*

You are probably going to need to take measures to stop the bleeding: birth control pills, Mirena IUD, or (if you are done having children) an endometrial ablation. Only then, will you be able to build your iron back up.

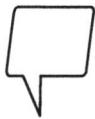

Anemia is only a symptom, telling you that you have to correct the blood loss. I was unable to raise my Hgb for a long time because I didn't stop the heavy bleeding. Finally, a good doctor told me that I was either going to have a blood transfusion or a procedure so I had the procedure, but not for about 6 months. Are you seeing your gynecologist?

I'm not sure what supplements you are on. Check the bottle and see how much elemental iron you are actually getting. For example; Ferris Sulfate has 326mgs but you are only getting 65 in that one dose. Even at two daily it's not really enough. You should ask your doctor about this to be sure. Especially considering your bleeding. My doctor told me that it was like having a hole in my bucket that cannot fill up.

These are some of the things that I learned through the course of my anemia. My Hgb would drop 1 point in 6 weeks. How is your Hgb holding up?

On the bright side of things as soon as I had my procedure my Hgb began to hold its own!

I have had low ferritin for years, but haven't done much, resisted iron due to side effects. Last year, I got some answers from reading about my hypothyroidism/Hashimoto's (hx=15 yrs) and how it can cause low ferritin, etc. I learned that I don't convert T4 to T3 and switched from synthetic T4 to Armour. I also found out I have adrenal fatigue. I learned that having a thyroid problem means I may have some vitamin/ mineral deficiencies. I started taking Adrenal Support, B's vitamins, magnesium, zinc, Wilsons Adrenal Stress Formula, Vitamin C, sea salt, floradix, sublingual ferrous sulfate (may stop- it is staining teeth), Iodoral, hydrocortisone, Vitamin D, fish oil. I feel SOOOO much better, except: significant hair loss and continued poor tolerance to exercise. I had labs done a couple of months ago and ferritin did not budge. I am thinking it is due to poor absorption. This is why we got a prescription for sublingual iron-but now I think it is staining my teeth. I am thinking of adding Betaine to help with absorption. Sound right?

Any input? Oh and I take C with my floradix. I may switch to Proferrin ES although that made me bloat- could that mean poor absorption? Would taking Betaine help? I am desperate to get my levels up. I hope to get in next week to draw labs. How many days to I stop the iron to get accurate test? Three days? Any other labs that would be helpful? I think I have a lot covered with the supplements. I use to only take levoxyl, now I take lots and feel so much better. This ferritin has me stumped though. I would love to STOP losing hair, it is scary.

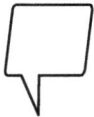

I'm not sure ****how much**** iron you are currently on. You do have to be on a good amount to raise your iron stores. Maybe this is your problem and not the absorption so much.

You don't have to worry so much about the iron and supplements because the ferritin is the true picture of iron stores and it is does not change results. The serum iron and sat% is changed but they usually don't do this one.

If you are concerned you can go off iron for 24 hrs, iron is rapidly absorbed from supplements and can skew the results of an iron study by making them falsely high.

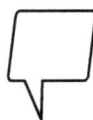

I'm in the same boat as you. Suffered with extremely low iron and took two years to raise it and that was when I found out that I had Hashimoto's.

A lot of thyroid sufferers have low iron problems. It is also very common for thyroid sufferers to have very low Vitamin D. Your doctor should check that also. Both iron and vitamin D malabsorbtion can be cause by gluten intolerance. Has anybody checked whether you are gluten intolerant? It's a simple blood test. Once again, we thyroid sufferers often have varying degrees of gluten intolerance.

With the vitamin D, when I was told to take it I began taking the basic 1000IU measurement (one gel capsule) as per instructions on the container. Next blood test I hadn't moved much and then my doctor issued me with some vitamin D drops which I drop 7 drops (4500IU) of onto my tongue each night after dinner. My vitamin D has moved up a little bit faster after taking a higher dosage. My doctor said taking vitamin D at night after dinner is more beneficial as it's more likely I would have eaten meat and the vitamin D absorbs better. Maybe this is due to the protein. He said vegetarians have a harder time absorbing vitamin D (and it has to be D3, not the other D).

I also have problems retaining iodine in my body. I lose more than I ought to and iodine is necessary for a healthy thyroid too.

I too have the adrenal issues. My doctor put me on Cortate tablets to help with my low morning cortisol levels and I'm so much better now. Are you only taking vitamin type supplements to help with your adrenals or are they actual medication what you are on?

If you were taking your iron along with the T4 you were on before that would make the T4 less effective and would also mean the T4 wouldn't be giving you the full benefit of making you feel better. You can take iron and other supplements alongside T3 medication's but not T4. I believe I was told to not take iron or other vitamins 2 hours prior and 4 hours after taking your T4 meds. This is going to worry me next week as I've only been on a T3 med (triiodothyronine) and as of Monday my doctor will be starting me on a little T4 (thyroxine). I'm juggling enough med's and supplements as it is and it frustrates me having to spread things out so that one thing doesn't inhibit another.

My medicinal listing and time frame is fast resembling a train time table It's ok if you are at *home all day, but I work full time and remembering and taking time out to take this, eat food prior to taking certain things, take one thing and wait before you can take another is driving me nuts. The thing is, nobody at work understands. They simply think thyroid issues are like a headache, you pop one pill and hey presto problem solved. They don't realize how much stuff I actually take and how tired I sometimes get. Maybe it's because I'm so good at hiding how I feel and just put on a happy face!!*

Just in case you didn't know, zinc should not be taken until either 2 hours prior or after taking your iron, just like caffeinated beverages, red wine and dairy products inhibit iron absorption.

Classification

Production vs. Destruction or Loss

The "kinetic" approach to anemia yields what many argue is the most clinically relevant classification of anemia. This classification depends on evaluation of several hematological parameters, particularly the blood reticulocyte (precursor of mature RBCs) count. This then yields the classification of defects by decreased RBC production versus increased RBC destruction and/or loss. Clinical signs of loss or destruction include abnormal peripheral blood smear with signs of hemolysis; elevated LDH suggesting cell destruction; or clinical signs of bleeding, such as guiaic-positive stool, radiographic findings, or frank bleeding.

Red Blood Cell Size

In the morphological approach, anemia is classified by the size of red blood cells; this is either done automatically or on microscopic examination of a peripheral blood smear. The size is reflected in the *mean corpuscular volume* (MCV). If the cells are smaller than normal (under 80 fl), the anemia is said to be *microcytic*; if they are normal size (80–100 fl), *normocytic*; and if they are larger than normal (over 100 fl), the anemia is classified as *macrocytic*. This scheme quickly exposes some of the most common causes of anemia; for instance, a microcytic anemia is often the result of iron deficiency. In clinical workup, the MCV will be one of the first pieces of information available; so even among clinicians who consider the "kinetic" approach more useful philosophically, morphology will remain an important element of classification and diagnosis.

Other characteristics visible on the peripheral smear may provide valuable clues about a more specific diagnosis; for example, abnormal white blood cells may point to a cause in the bone marrow.

Microcytic Anemia

Microcytic anemia is primarily a result of hemoglobin synthesis failure/insufficiency, which could be caused by several etiologies:

- Heme synthesis defect
  - Iron deficiency anemia
  - Anemia of chronic disease (more commonly presenting as normocytic anemia)
- Globin synthesis defect
  - alpha-, and beta-thalassemia
  - HbE syndrome
  - HbC syndrome
  - and various other unstable hemoglobin diseases
- Sideroblastic defect
  - Hereditary sideroblastic anemia
  - Acquired sideroblastic anemia, including lead toxicity
  - Reversible sideroblastic anemia

Iron deficiency anemia is the most common type of anemia overall and it has many causes. RBCs often appear hypochromic (paler than usual) and microcytic (smaller than usual) when viewed with a microscope.

- Iron deficiency anemia is caused by insufficient dietary intake or absorption of iron to replace losses from menstruation or losses due to diseases.[11] Iron is an essential part of hemoglobin, and low iron levels result in decreased incorporation of hemoglobin into red blood cells. In the United States, 20% of all women of childbearing age have iron deficiency anemia, compared with only 2% of adult men. The principal cause of iron deficiency anemia in premenopausal women is blood lost during menses. Studies have shown that iron deficiency without anemia causes poor school performance and lower IQ in teenage girls. Iron deficiency is the most prevalent deficiency state on a worldwide basis. Iron deficiency is sometimes the cause of abnormal fissuring of the angular (corner) sections of the lips (angular stomatitis).

- Iron deficiency anemia can also be due to bleeding lesions of the gastrointestinal tract. Fecal occult blood testing, upper endoscopy and lower endoscopy should be performed to identify bleeding lesions. In men and post-menopausal women the chances are higher that bleeding from the gastrointestinal tract could be due to colon polyp or colorectal cancer.

• Worldwide, the most common cause of iron deficiency anemia is parasitic infestation (hookworm, amebiasis, schistosomiasis and whipworm).[12]

Macrocytic Anemia

• Megaloblastic anemia, the most common cause of macrocytic anemia, is due to a deficiency of either vitamin B-12, folic acid (or both). Deficiency in folate and/or vitamin B-12 can be due either to inadequate intake or insufficient absorption. Folate deficiency normally does not produce neurological symptoms, while B-12 deficiency does.

  • Pernicious anemia is caused by a lack of intrinsic factor. Intrinsic factor is required to absorb vitamin B-12 from food. A lack of intrinsic factor may arise from an autoimmune condition targeting the parietal cells (atrophic gastritis) that produce intrinsic factor or against intrinsic factor itself. These lead to poor absorption of vitamin B-12.

- Macrocytic anemia can also be caused by removal of the functional portion of the stomach, such as during gastric bypass surgery, leading to reduced vitamin B-12/folate absorption. Therefore one must always be aware of anemia following this procedure.

- Hypothyroidism

- Alcoholism commonly causes a macrocytosis, although not specifically anemia. Other types of Liver Disease can also cause macrocytosis.

- Methotrexate, zidovudine, and other drugs that inhibit DNA replication.

Macrocytic anemia can be further divided into "megaloblastic anemia" or "non-megaloblastic macrocytic anemia". The cause of megaloblastic anemia is primarily a failure of DNA synthesis with preserved RNA synthesis, which results in restricted cell division of the progenitor cells. The megaloblastic anemias often present with neutrophil hypersegmentation (6–10 lobes). The non-megaloblastic macrocytic anemias have different etiologies (i.e. there is unimpaired DNA globin synthesis,) which occur, for example in alcoholism.

In addition to the non-specific symptoms of anemia, specific features of vitamin B-12 deficiency include peripheral neuropathy and subacute combined degeneration of the cord with resulting balance difficulties from posterior column spinal cord pathology.[13] Other features may include a smooth, red tongue and glossitis.

The treatment for vitamin B-12-deficient anemia was first devised by William Murphy who bled dogs to make them anemic and then fed them various substances to see what (if anything) would make them healthy again. He discovered that ingesting large amounts of liver seemed to cure the disease. George Minot and George Whipple then set about to chemically isolate the curative substance and ultimately were able to isolate the vitamin B-12 from the liver. All three shared the 1934 Nobel Prize in Medicine.[14]

Is pernicious anemia hereditary? My mother is dead and I'm unable to ask her.

Yes, it is classed as an autoimmune disease. It does suggest a hereditary component.

Pernicious anemia happens when the destruction of the gastric cells no longer have the ability to make (IF) intrinsic factor. IF is what helps B-12 to be absorbed by the intestines which can cause B-12 deficiency.

If you think that you have this you should also be checked for H-Pylor bacteria, they *think* that there may be an association linked.

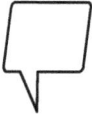

Here is a list of the tests doctors use to diagnose pernicious anemia:

- *Via blood tests--H-pylori. Intrinsic factorand Parietal Cell antibody tests are normally done.*
- *Also, markers for B-12 deficiency include Methylmalonic acid (MMA) and Homocysteine which can be elevated in PA.*

These tests are used to rule out and diagnose pernicious anemia focus on finding a cause for cobalamine def. Many times these tests are done in stages and IF may be the first to be tested.

Normocytic Anemia

Normocytic anemia occurs when the overall hemoglobin levels are always decreased, but the red blood cell size (Mean corpuscular volume) remains normal. Causes include:

- Acute blood loss

- Anemia of chronic disease

- Aplastic anemia (bone marrow failure)

- Hemolytic anemia

I learned something interesting while researching inflammation that may help explain the difference between anemia of chronic inflammation and anemia of chronic renal failure.

Inflammation greatly contributes to the anemia of chronic renal failure by restricting the bone marrow's responsiveness to the endogenous hormone erythropoietin and ESA therapy.

Both anemia of chronic disease (aka chronic inflammation) and anemia of renal failure (CRF) result in a decreased production of red blood cells. Both are classified as normochromic and normocytic anemias. Anemia of CRF is thought to result mainly from a combination of erythropoietin deficiency and anemia of chronic disease. It is more severe than other forms of anemia and often leads to cardiovascular complications. This type of anemia also contributes to cerebrovascular diseases, poor muscle strength, fatigue and decreased mobility.

The main cause of anemia of CRF is an impaired production of erythropoietin hormone in the kidneys. Often, there are other contributing factors, such as an abnormal absorption and use of iron, so typical in anemia of inflammation. The two conditions are very closely linked. I read that it is possible for a person with anemia of CRF to develop anemia of inflammation.

Anemia of CRF does not respond to iron, folate or vitamin B-12 supplementation. It is usually treated with synthetic erythropoietin stimulating agents (ESAs). Interestingly, the target hemoglobin level range in people with chronic kidney disease is only 11–12 g/Dl. Higher hemoglobin values are likely to cause harm.

Dimorphic Anemia

When two causes of anemia act simultaneously, e.g., macrocytic hypochromic, due to hookworm infestation leading to deficiency of both iron and vitamin B-12 or folic acid[15] or following a blood transfusion more than one abnormality of red cell indices may be seen. Evidence for multiple causes appears with an elevated RBC distribution width (RDW), which suggests a wider-than-normal range of red cell sizes.

Heinz Body Anemia

Heinz bodies form in the cytoplasm of RBCs and appear like small dark dots under the microscope. There are many causes of Heinz body anemia, and some forms can be drug induced. It is triggered in cats by eating onions[16] or acetaminophen (Tylenol). It can be triggered in dogs by ingesting onions or zinc, and in horses by ingesting dry red maple leaves.

Specific Anemias

• Anemia of prematurity occurs in premature infants at 2–6 weeks of age and results from diminished erythropoietin response to declining hematocrit levels.

• Aplastic anemia is a condition generally unresponsive to anti-anemia therapies where bone marrow fails to produce enough red blood cells.

• Fanconi anemia is a hereditary disorder or defect featuring aplastic anemia and various other abnormalities.

• Hemolytic anemia causes a separate constellation of symptoms (also featuring jaundice and elevated LDH levels) with numerous potential causes. It can be autoimmune, immune, hereditary or mechanical (e.g. heart surgery). It can result (because of cell fragmentation) in a microcytic anemia, a normochromic anemia, or (because of premature release of immature red blood cells from the bone marrow), a macrocytic anemia.

- Hereditary spherocytosis is a hereditary defect that results in defects in the RBC cell membrane, causing the erythrocytes to be sequestered and destroyed by the spleen. This leads to a decrease in the number of circulating RBCs and, hence, anemia.

- Sickle-cell anemia, a hereditary disorder, is due to homozygous hemoglobin S genes.

- Warm autoimmune hemolytic anemia is an anemia caused by autoimmune attack against red blood cells, primarily by IgG.

- Cold agglutinin hemolytic anemia is primarily mediated by IgM.

- Pernicious anemia is a form of megaloblastic anemia due to vitamin B-12 deficiency dependent on impaired absorption of vitamin B-12.

- Myelophthisic anemia or Myelophthisis is a severe type of anemia resulting from the replacement of bone marrow by other materials, such as malignant tumors or granulomas.

- Anemia of Pregnancy is anemia that is induced by blood volume expansion experienced in pregnancy.

Possible Complications

Anemia diminishes the capability of individuals who are affected to perform physical activities. This is a result of one's muscles being forced to depend on anaerobic metabolism. The lack of iron associated with anemia can cause many complications, including hypoxemia, brittle or rigid fingernails, cold intolerance, and possible behavioral disturbances in children. Hypoxemia resulting from anemia can worsen the cardio-pulmonary status of patients with pre-existing chronic pulmonary disease. Cold intolerance occurs in one in five patients with iron deficiency anemia, and becomes visible through numbness and tingling.

Anemia during Pregnancy

Anemia affects 20% of all females of childbearing age in the United States. Because of the subtlety of the symptoms, women are often unaware that they have this disorder, as they attribute the symptoms to the stresses of their daily lives. Possible problems for the fetus include increased risk of growth retardation, prematurity, intrauterine death, rupture of the amnion and infection.

During pregnancy, women should be especially aware of the symptoms of anemia, as an adult female loses an average of two milligrams of iron daily. Therefore, she must intake a similar quantity of iron in order to make up for this loss. Additionally, a woman loses approximately 500 milligrams of iron with each pregnancy, compared with a loss of 4–100 milligrams of iron with each period. Possible consequences for the mother include cardiovascular symptoms, reduced physical and mental performance, reduced immune function, fatigue, reduced peripartal blood reserves and increased need for blood transfusion in the postpartum period.

Does anyone know the possible effects of being anaemic whilst pregnant and breast feeding on the child?

Could it affect their health? What do we need to look out for, if anything?

Do you know of any research?

While breast milk is rich in antibodies, it is poor in iron. A study found the link between low levels of iron in blood of breastfeeding women and higher risk of anemia in their babies. I would think that thing to do is regular checkups with the pediatrician, and your regular checkups for CBC and anemia.

My daughter is five now but she constantly looks pale, she is a great eater and eats all kinds of fruit and vegetables but is picking up lots of infections (which means lots of time off for me which is not good). So I wonder... if I was anaemic when pregnant with her and also whilst breast feeding if this may have had an effect on her... ???

Well, that may have resolved if it did happen after she started on solid foods. Anemia can be resolved through diet alone, believe it or not if there isn't an underlying condition and all is well.

In your daughter's case it is common for small children to be low in iron or even to be anemic. This is due to the increase of demand for iron due to growth spurts and possibly diets low in iron.

Treatments for Anemia

There are many different treatments for anemia and the treatment depends on severity and the cause.

Iron deficiency from nutritional causes is rare in non-menstruating adults (men and post-menopausal women). The diagnosis of iron deficiency mandates a search for potential sources of loss such as gastrointestinal bleeding from ulcers or colon cancer. Mild to moderate iron deficiency anemia is treated by iron supplementation with ferrous sulfate or ferrous gluconate. Vitamin C may aid in the body's ability to absorb iron.

Vitamin supplements given orally (folic acid) or subcutaneously (vitamin B-12) will replace specific deficiencies.

In anemia of chronic disease, anemia associated with chemotherapy, or anemia associated with renal disease, some clinicians prescribe recombinant erythropoietin, epoetin alfa, to stimulate red cell production.

In severe cases of anemia, or with ongoing blood loss, a blood transfusion may be necessary.

I have anemia for iron deficiency , The doctor told me to take iron pills I tried I think everything in pills I doesn't work , I had problems in my stomach (nausea, diarrhea, cramps), there are other pills to take without have problems in my stomach?

There are many types of iron that you can try. I take Poly Iron 150. I cannot take Ferris Sulfate or anything (iron salts based) like that at all. I get mine without a script from within the pharmacy behind the counter. You should ask your doctor for a gastrointestinal friendly iron or you can talk to your pharmacist about things that you can ask your doctor for.

I had the same problem as you with iron causing diarrhea. I now take amino chelated iron and I don't have any problems with it.

Blood Transfusions for Anemia

Doctors attempt to avoid blood transfusion in general, since multiple lines of evidence point to increased adverse patient clinical outcomes with more intensive transfusion strategies. The physiological principle that reduction of oxygen delivery associated with anemia leads to adverse clinical outcomes is balanced by the finding that transfusion does not necessarily mitigate these adverse clinical outcomes.

In severe, acute bleeding, transfusions of donated blood are often lifesaving. Improvements in battlefield casualty survival is attributable, at least in part, to the recent improvements in blood banking and transfusion techniques.

Transfusion of the stable but anemic hospitalized patient has been the subject of numerous clinical trials, and transfusion is emerging as a deleterious intervention.

Four randomized controlled clinical trials have been conducted to evaluate aggressive versus conservative transfusion strategies in critically ill patients. All four of these studies failed to find a benefit with more aggressive transfusion strategies.[17][18][19][20]

In addition, at least two retrospective studies have shown increases in adverse clinical outcomes with more aggressive transfusion strategies.[21][22]

Hyperbaric Oxygenation

Treatment of exceptional blood loss (anemia) is recognized as an indication for hyperbaric oxygen (HBO) by the Undersea and Hyperbaric Medical Society.[23][24] The use of HBO is indicated when oxygen delivery to tissue is not sufficient in patients who cannot be transfused for medical or religious reasons. HBO may be used for medical reasons when threat of blood product incompatibility or concern for transmissible disease are factors.[23] The beliefs of some religions (ex: Jehovah's Witnesses) may prohibit the receipt of transfused blood products.[23]

In 2002, Van Meter reviewed the publications surrounding the use of HBO in severe anemia and found that all publications report a positive result.[25]

My son is 14 weeks old, six weeks old adjusted age (he was eight weeks early). Due to being premature and therefore more likely to have low iron, we had his iron levels checked through a blood draw. His hemoglobin came back at 8.5, but his ferritin levels were normal. It is my understanding that normal ferritin levels mean that he has normal iron stores, and therefore is not low on iron but the low hemoglobin indicates his body is not using the iron it has. Is this correct? The pediatrician recommended we start my son on iron supplements but is that really THE best course of action? What can cause low hemoglobin when ferritin levels are normal?

You could always try the iron supplements for a short course and then have the hemoglobin checked again to see if it is working, say in 4–6 weeks. If it's not working you can go from there.

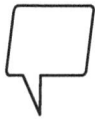

There is nothing to worry about. This is a normal physiologic process that occurs in all newborns but in premature infants, the drop in Hgb occurs a little earlier and is greater. Preemies drop their Hgb to about 8 gm/dL around the 4–8 week mark. Full term infants drop to an average of 11.5 gm dL, by 6–10 weeks. This phenomenon is called nadir. The drop does not occur because of lack of iron stores, instead the production of red blood cells drops off to allow the infant to adapt to life outside the uterus. This is referred to as the reticulocyte production and it drops from 6–10% down to - 1%, by five days of age. Your baby's Hgb actually reflects that he is starting to climb back up from his lowest point. Your pediatrician should have explained this to you so as not to cause you undue worry. Give your son the iron, as prescribed. Good luck and enjoy your little miracle.

If it is a normal occurrence, then why does he need the supplemental iron? I am okay with giving it to him if he needs it, but if he doesn't need it then I don't want to. If he was older I would be less hesitant but he is still very young with an open gut. If the levels are going back up on their own, what good will the supplemental iron do? What harm is there if I don't give it to *him and we keep a close eye on his levels to make sure they aren't going down?*

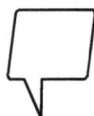

Your first question about whether the iron supplementation is required really depends on what you are feeding your son. Is he breastfed or receiving formula? Breastfed babies generally require no extra iron supplementation. Some formulas have iron but some don't. Most pediatricians will prescribe iron if your baby is receiving a formula that does not contain iron.

The second issue is that preemies are more prone to iron deficiency anemia. The fetus receives its iron stores from his mother during the last trimester of pregnancy. If the baby comes too early, then he did not receive that store of iron that should maintain them through their first six months. Once babies start to eat solids, they often will take an iron supplementation. Solid baby foods are often low in iron.

I would, definitely, voice your concerns to your pediatrician and make a decision together. I don't know all of your baby's medical history but your doctor does and he would have a much better idea of what your little guy needs. If you would rather take a wait and see attitude, let your doctor know.

If you want to read more about the natural drop in Hgb in infants, just type these into a search engine and you will get many hits.

MEGALOBLASTIC ANEMIA

Megaloblastic anemia is an anemia (of macrocytic classification) which results from inhibition of DNA synthesis in red blood cell production.[1] This is often due to deficiency of vitamin B-12 and/or folic acid. Megaloblastic anemia not due to hypovitaminosis may be caused by antimetabolites which poison DNA production, such as some chemotherapeutic or antimicrobial agents (for example azathioprine or trimethoprim).

It is characterized by many large immature and dysfunctional red blood cells (megaloblasts) in the bone marrow,[2] and also by hypersegmented or multisegmented neutrophils.

Causes

• Vitamin B-12 deficiency:

  • achlorhydria-induced malabsorption

  • Deficient intake

  • Deficient intrinsic factor (pernicious anemia or gastrectomy)

- Biological competition for B-12 by diverticulosis, fistula, intestinal anastomosis, and infection by the marine parasite Diphyllobothrium latum

- Selective B-12 malabsorption (congenital and drug-induced)

- Chronic pancreatitis

- Ileal resection and bypass

- Nitrous oxyde anaesthesis

- Folate deficiency:

  - alcoholism

  - Deficient intake.

  - Increased needs: pregnancy, infant, rapid cellular proliferation, and cirrhosis

  - Malabsorption (congenital and drug-induced)

  - Intestinal and jujenal resection

- Combined Deficiency (Tropical sprue): Vitamin B-12 and Folate.

- Inherited Pyrimidine Synthesis Disorders: Orotic Aciduria

- Inherited DNA Synthesis Disorders: Deficient thiamine and factors (e.g. enzymes) responsible for folate metabolism.

- Toxins and Drugs:

  - Folic acid antagonists (methotrexate)

  - Purine synthesis antagonists (6-mercaptopurine)

  - Pyrimidine antagonists (cytosine arabinoside)

  - Phenytoin

- Erythroleukemia

Hematological Findings

The blood film can point towards vitamin deficiency:

- Decreased red blood cell (RBC) count and hemoglobin levels

- Increased mean corpuscular volume (MCV, >95 fl) and mean corpuscular hemoglobin (MCH)

- Normal mean corpuscular hemoglobin concentration (MCHC, 32–36 g/dL)

- The reticulocyte count is decreased due to destruction of fragile and abnormal megaloblastic erythroid precursor.

- The platelet count may be reduced.

- Neutrophil granulocytes may show multisegmented nuclei ("senile neutrophil"). This is thought to be due to decreased production and a compensatory prolonged lifespan for circulating neutrophils, which increase numbers of nuclear segments with age.

- Anisocytosis (increased variation in RBC size) and poikilocytosis (abnormally shaped RBCs).

- Macrocytes (larger than normal RBCs) are present.

- Ovalocytes (oval-shaped RBCs) are present.

- Howell-Jolly bodies (chromosomal remnant) also present.

Blood chemistries will also show:

- Increased homocysteine and methylmalonic acid in B-12 deficiency

- Increased homocysteine in folate deficiency

Normal levels of both methylmalonic acid and total homocysteine rule out clinically significant cobalamin deficiency with virtual certainty.[3]

Bone marrow (not normally checked in a patient suspected of megaloblastic anemia) shows megaloblastic hyperplasia.

Possible Associated Neurological Findings

Subacute combined degeneration of spinal cord and its symptoms may be present, due to demyelination secondary to deficiency of vitamin B-12.

Analysis

The gold standard for the diagnosis of B-12 deficiency is a low blood level of B-12. A low level of blood B-12 is a symptom which normally can and should be treated by injections, supplementation, or dietary or lifestyle advice, but it is not a diagnosis. Hypovitaminosis B-12 can result from a number of mechanisms, including those listed above. For determination of etiology, further patient history, testing, and empirical therapy may be clinically indicated.

A measurement of methylmalonic acid can provide an indirect method for partially differentiating B-12 and folate deficiencies. The level of methylmalonic acid is not elevated in folic acid deficiency. But direct measurement of blood cobalamin remains the gold standard because the test for elevated methylmalonic acid is not specific enough. Vitamin B-12 is one necessary prosthetic group to the enzyme methylmalonyl-coenzyme A mutase. B-12 deficiency is but one among the conditions that can lead to dysfunction of this enzyme and a buildup of its substrate, methylmalonic acid, the elevated level of which can be detected in the urine and blood.

Due to the lack of available radioactive B-12, the Schilling test is now largely a historical artifact. The Schilling test was performed in the past to help determine the nature of the vitamin B-12 deficiency. An advantage of the Schilling test was that it often included B-12 with intrinsic factor.

IRON DEFICIENCY ANEMIA

Iron deficiency anemia is the common type of anemia, and is also known as sideropenic anemia. It is the most common cause of microcytic anemia.

Iron deficiency anemia occurs when the dietary intake or absorption of iron is insufficient, and hemoglobin, which contains iron, cannot be formed.[1] In the United States, 20% of all women of childbearing age have iron deficiency anemia, compared with only 2% of adult men. The principal cause of iron deficiency anemia in premenopausal women is blood lost during menses. Iron deficiency anemia can be caused by parasitic infections, such as hookworms. Intestinal bleeding caused by hookworms can lead to fecal blood loss and heme/iron deficiency.[2] Chronic inflammation caused by parasitic infections contributes to anemia during pregnancy in most developing countries.[3]

Iron deficiency anemia is an advanced stage of iron deficiency. When the body has sufficient iron to meet its needs (functional iron), the remainder is stored for later use in the bone marrow, liver, and spleen as part of a finely tuned system of human iron metabolism. Iron deficiency ranges from iron depletion, which yields little physiological damage, to iron deficiency anemia, which can affect the function of numerous organ systems. Iron depletion causes the amount of stored iron to be reduced, but has no effect on the functional iron. However, a person with no stored iron has no reserves to use if the body requires more iron. In essence, the amount of iron absorbed and stored by the body is not adequate for growth and development or to replace the amount lost.

What are the differences between anemia of chronic disease/chronic inflammation and anemia secondary to chronic kidney disease? How could an individual with chronic inflammation, chronic kidney disease and an iron deficiency determine the type of anemia he/she has? Is there a way to make this distinction through labwork? Things could get somewhat complicated if the anemia was an end result of several abnormalities.

The text I read mentioned that the anemia of chronic disease/inflammation and anemia secondary to chronic kidney disease share some characteristics, without being specific. I am surprised to learn that they are two distinct conditions.

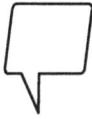

Anemia of chronic disease is when you have inflammation, cancer, autoimmune diseases, and such that result in anemia. Usually, they are mild to moderate and when treated the anemia may be resolved or kept at mild levels.

Anemia secondary to chronic kidney disease is when anemia is a result of just that; chronic kidney disease (CKD), EPO's and then there is iron deficiency that can coexist on top of that.

History

A disease believed to be iron deficiency anemia is described in about 1500 B.C. in the Egyptian Ebers papyrus. It was termed *chlorosis* or *green sickness* in Medieval Europe, and iron salts were used for treatment in France by the mid-17th century. Thomas Sydenham recommended iron salts as treatment for chlorosis, but treatment with iron was controversial until the 20th century, when its mechanism of action was more fully elucidated.

Symptoms

Iron deficiency anemia is characterized by pallor (reduced amount of oxyhemoglobin in skin or mucous membrane), fatigue and weakness. Because it tends to develop slowly, adaptation occurs and the disease often goes unrecognized for some time. In severe cases, dyspnea (trouble breathing) can occur. Unusual obsessive food cravings, known as pica, may develop. Pagophagia or pica for ice is a very specific symptom and may disappear with correction of iron deficiency anemia. Hair loss and lightheadedness can also be associated with iron deficiency anemia.

Just wondering how long the hair shedding lasts typically. I still notice quite a bit of hair loss. Last I checked (three months ago) my iron was just getting into normal range. I just got my blood checked recently and am waiting to get thru to the doctor to get the results.

To my knowledge, I've been dealing with low iron for almost two years know. I'm feeling better so I assume that my iron is better... however I still have hair loss?

I'm beginning to think that my thyroid might have something to do with my situation but I've had it tested many times and to my knowledge it's fine.

This is very different for everyone. My hair has always done a little shedding throughout the years. I probably had hypothyroidism at the time and never knew it. I, like you, and many others also had low iron for many years prior to my illness and diagnosis. My hair started falling out really bad to where I could notice a difference in the amount and new hairs all over my head. When my ferritin got to 20 I noticed that it slowed way down and only got better from there.

When it comes to your thyroid, this can change at any given moment, so you may want to check it out again. I have mine checked every three months, but I have Hashimoto's.

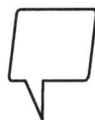

Your hair loss is, unfortunately, most likely may be due to your genetics.

Chronic iron deficiency

Symptoms
- Rapid hair loss
- Weight loss
- Pale appearance
- Spoon-shaped nails
- Depression
- Change of hair color to a lighter shade
- Excessive dryness of hair

Causes

- *Vitamin C deficiency , which can also lead to an iron deficiency*
- *Heavy consumption of caffeine rich tea and coffee since caffeine reduces the net availability of iron supplied through food.*
- *Alcohol abuse also reduces the availability of iron in the body .Even slightly low levels of iron can cause diffuse hair loss.*

Sources

- *Rice, bread, broccoli and beans.*
- *Vitamin C is required for good absorption.*

Anemia due to copper deficiency, known as copper deficiency anemia

Copper besides acting as catalyst in oxidation of hydrogen and the formation of melanin (the pigment that gives hair its color), is also needed to release iron stored in liver, for intestinal absorption of iron into the hemoglobin.

Sources: Mushrooms, grains, nuts, beans.

Other Symptoms

Other symptoms patients with iron deficiency anemia have reported are:

- Constipation
- Sleepiness
- Tinnitus
- Palpitations
- Seeing bright colors
- Fainting or feeling faint
- Depression
- Breathlessness
- Twitching muscles
- Tingling, numbness, or burning sensations
- Sleep apnea (rare)
- Missed menstrual cycle
- Heavy menstrual period
- Slow social development
- Glossitis
- Angular chelitis
- Koilonychia (spoon-shaped nails) or nails that are weak or brittle

- Poor appetite

- Pruritus

I was recently diagnosed with anemia with a very low red blood cell count of 8. I have fibroids and very heavy periods, so I guess that explains it. I've been on the iron tabs (250mg x 3 a day) for three days and felt great for two days, but today I feel too tired to do anything and the shaking, heart palpitations, sore throat, dry mouth and general flu-like symptoms have returned.

The weirdest thing has been the burning sensations - and I understand it can be a side effect of iron deficiency to get burning and soreness in the hands and feet and also the tongue, but I can't find it documented anywhere that you can also get burning and stinging in the genital area.

My doctor took a swab which was clear and I have no other symptoms (e.g. discharge, etc). Everything else is normal and this is not thrush as I previously thought. It is definitely related to the anemia because it almost went away over the last two days and then was back yesterday evening, but this time just externally rather than inside my vagina, which had been the case before. It is excruciating and the only thing that calms it down is yoghurt (I guess because it has a cooling effect). It also only gets really bad in the evening and then in the morning, after sleep, it feels ok again.

I've heard that occasionally this can be a symptom of pernicious anemia (B-12 deficiency), but not of iron deficiency.

Has anyone else experienced this, or heard about it - please let me know because both I and my doctor are baffled by this, and it's also quite scary.

The burning, especially vaginally, wouldn't be pleasant. So long as your doctor has taken swabs and checked for all things possible. It could be a light case of yeast or bacterial vaginosis. Maybe if you post on the Women's Health section of the boards. Someone there might have more experience in that area.

I'm amazed. I've kept a list of my weird sensations, and they include yours. It all started after Serotonin Syndrome and Serotonin Withdrawal. I've had burning/stinging sensations in my groin, hands, feet, brain, and mouth. The burning in my groin and hands is almost gone, but in the mouth, feet, and brain it's still very strong. I haven't gotten any help from doctors. I did get a B-12 shot a couple of weeks ago, but nothing has changed. I've had CT and MRI, and showed no abnormalities. I have problems at C-5/6 and C-6/7, but so do lots of folks. I was amazed to find people having these same sensations.

Is it normal for symptoms to come and go when you're recovering? Sometimes I feel OK, although always tired, and other days I get the fast heart beat and shaking and chest pain or the burning sensations, then they go away again. No two days have been the same.

I'm also extremely worried about getting my period. I have period pain at the moment and this can last a week before my period comes. I'm really concerned the burning and other symptoms will get worse again through the loss of blood and I'll have to start from scratch. The doctor gave me some Melanefic Acid or something which is an anti-inflammatory to help with period pain and hopefully make my period less heavy, but she says it may or may not work.

If I'm on the iron tabs will my period make a lot of difference to my recovery in your experience?

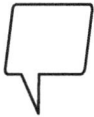

I'm responding to your comment about period pain a week before your period starts.

I had endometriosis and had terrible pain before my period. Also knew when I ovulated because that was painful too. Have you mentioned this to your gynecologist?

I'm sure endometriosis can cause anemia too, because it is abnormal bleeding. I had it over 25 years ago and not much was known about it then- but I think it is well understood today.

Infant Development

Iron deficiency anemia for infants in their earlier stages of development may have significantly greater consequences than it does for adults. An animal made severely iron deficient during its earlier life cannot recover to normal iron levels even with iron therapy. In contrast, iron deficiency during later stages of development can be compensated with sufficient iron supplements. Iron deficiency anemia affects neurological development by decreasing learning ability, altering motor functions, and permanently reducing the number of dopamine receptors and serotonin levels. Iron deficiency during development can lead to reduced myelination of the spinal cord, as well as a change in myelin composition. Additionally, iron deficiency anemia has a negative effect on physical growth. Growth hormone secretion is related to serum transferrin levels, suggesting a positive correlation between iron-transferrin levels and an increase in height and weight.

Diagnosis

Anemia may be diagnosed from symptoms and signs, but when anemia is mild it may not be diagnosed from mild non-specific symptoms. Anemia is often first shown by routine blood tests, which generally include a complete blood count (CBC). A sufficiently low hemoglobin (HGB) or hematocrit (HCT) value is characteristic of anemia, and further studies will be undertaken to determine its cause and the exact diagnosis. One of the first abnormal values to be noted on a CBC will be a high red blood cell distribution width (RDW), reflecting a varied size distribution of red blood cells (RBCs). A low MCV, MCH or MCHC, and the appearance of the RBCs on visual examination of a peripheral blood smear will narrow the diagnosis to a *microcytic anemia*. The blood smear of a patient with iron deficiency shows many hypochromatic and rather small RBCs, and may also show poikilocytosis (variation in shape) and anisocytosis (variation in size), and a few target cells. Microcytic anemia can also be the result of malabsorption phenomena associated with gluten-sensitive enteropathy/coeliac disease.

The diagnosis of iron deficiency anemia will be suggested by appropriate history (e.g., anemia in a menstruating woman), and by such diagnostic tests as a low serum ferritin, a low serum iron level, an elevated serum transferrin and a high total iron binding capacity (TIBC). Serum ferritin is the most sensitive lab test for iron deficiency anemia.

Change in lab values in iron deficiency anemia	
Change	Parameter
Decrease	ferritin, hemoglobin, MCV
Increase	TIBC, transferrin, RDW

Iron deficient anemia and thalassemia minor present with many of the same lab results. It is very important not to treat a patient with thalassemia with an iron supplement as this can lead to hemachromatosis (accumulation of iron in the liver). A hemoglobin electrophoresis would provide useful evidence in distinguishing these two conditions, along with iron studies.

> *My son is 14 weeks old, six weeks old adjusted age (he was eight weeks early). Due to being premature and therefore more likely to have low iron, we had his iron levels checked through a blood draw. His hemoglobin came back at 8.5, but his ferritin levels were normal. It is my understanding that normal ferritin levels mean that he has normal iron stores, and therefore is not low on iron but the low hemoglobin indicates his body is not using the iron it has. Is this correct? The pediatrician recommended we start my son on iron supplements but is that really THE best course of action? What can cause low hemoglobin when ferritin levels are normal?*

> *You could always try the iron supplements for a short course and then have the hemoglobin checked again to see if it is working, say in 4–6 weeks. If it's not working, you can go from there.*

> *There is nothing to worry about. This is a normal physiologic process that occurs in all newborns but in premature infants, the drop in Hgb occurs a little earlier and is greater. Preemies drop their Hgb to about 8 gm/dL around the 4–8 week mark. Full*

term infants drop to an average of 11.5 gm dL, by 6–10 weeks. This phenomenon is called nadir. The drop does not occur because of lack of iron stores, instead the production of red blood cells drops off to allow the infant to adapt to life outside the uterus. This is referred to as the reticulocyte production and it drops from 6–10% down to - 1%, by five days of age. Your baby's Hgb actually reflects that he is starting to climb back up from his lowest point. Your pediatrician should have explained this to you so as not to cause you undue worry. Give your son the iron, as prescribed. Good luck and enjoy your little miracle.

If it is a normal occurrence, then why does he need the supplemental iron? I am okay with giving it to him if he needs it, but if he doesn't need it then I don't want to. If he was older I would be less hesitant but he is still very young with an open gut. If the levels are going back up on their own, what good will the supplemental iron do? What harm is there if I don't give it to him and we keep a close eye on his levels to make sure they aren't going down?

Great questions. Your first question about whether the iron supplementation is required really depends on what you are feeding your son. Is he breastfed or receiving formula? Breastfed babies generally require no extra iron supplementation. Some formulas have iron but some don't. Most pediatricians will prescribe iron if your baby is receiving a formula that does not contain iron.

The second issue is that preemies are more prone to iron deficiency anemia. The fetus receives its iron stores from his mother during the last trimester of pregnancy. If the baby comes too early, then he did not receive that store of iron that should maintain them through their first six months. Once babies start to eat solids, they often will take a iron supplementation. Solid baby foods are often low in iron.

I would, definitely, voice your concerns to your pediatrician and make a decision together. I don't know all of your baby's medical history but your doctor does and he would have a much better idea of what your little guy needs. If you would rather take a wait and see attitude, let you doctor know.

If you want to read more about the natural drop in Hgb in infants, just type these into a search engine and you will get many hits.

Gold Standard

Traditionally, a definitive diagnosis requires a demonstration of depleted body iron stores by performing a bone marrow aspiration, with the marrow stained for iron.[4][5] Because this is invasive and painful, while a clinical trial of iron supplementation is inexpensive and non-traumatic, patients are often treated based on clinical history and serum ferritin levels without a bone marrow biopsy. Furthermore, a study published April 2009[6] questions the value of stainable bone marrow iron following parenteral iron therapy.

Determination of Etiology

The diagnosis of iron deficiency anemia requires further investigation as to its cause. It can be a sign of other disease, such as colon cancer, which will cause the loss of blood in the stool. In adults, 60% of patients with iron deficiency anemia may have underlying gastrointestinal disorders leading to chronic blood loss. In addition to dietary insufficiency, malabsorption, chronic blood loss, diversion of iron to fetal erythropoiesis during pregnancy, intravascular haemolysis and haemoglobinuria or other forms of chronic blood loss should all be considered.

Treatment

If the cause is dietary iron deficiency, iron supplements, usually with iron (II) sulfate, ferrous gluconate, or iron amino acid chelate ferrous bisglycinate, synthetic chelate NaFerredetate, EDTA will usually correct the anemia.

Recent research suggests the replacement dose of iron, at least in the elderly with iron deficiency, may be as little as 15 mg per day of elemental iron. An experiment done in a group of 130 anemia patients showed a 98% increase in iron count when using an iron supplement with an average of 100 mg of iron. Women who develop iron deficiency anemia in mid-pregnancy can be effectively treated with low doses of iron (20–40 mg per day). The lower dose is effective and produces fewer gastrointestinal complaints.

Many tests have shown that iron supplementation can lead to an increase in infectious disease morbidity in areas where bacterial infections are common. For example, children receiving iron-enriched foods have demonstrated an increased rate in diarrhea overall and enteropathogen shedding. Iron deficiency protects against infection by creating an unfavorable environment for bacterial growth. Nevertheless, while iron deficiency might lessen infections by certain pathogenic diseases, it also leads to a reduction in resistance to other strains of viral or bacterial infections, such as *Salmonella typhimurium* or *Entamoeba histolytica*. Overall, it may be concluded that iron supplementation can be both beneficial and harmful to an individual in an environment that is prone to many infectious diseases.

There can be a great difference between iron intake and iron absorption, also known as bioavailability. Scientific studies indicate iron absorption problems when iron is taken in conjunction with milk, tea, coffee and other substances. There are already a number of proven solutions for this problem, including:

- Fortification with ascorbic acid, which increases bioavailability in both presence and absence of inhibiting substances, but which is subject to deterioration from moisture or heat. Ascorbic acid fortification is usually limited to sealed dried foods, but individuals can easily take ascorbic acid with basic iron supplement for the same benefits.

- Microencapsulation with lecithin, which binds and protects the iron particles from the action of inhibiting substances. The primary benefit over ascorbic acid is durability and shelf life, particularly for products like milk which undergo heat treatment.

- Using an iron amino acid chelate, such as NaFeEDTA, which similarly binds and protects the iron particles. A study performed by the Hematology Unit of the University of Chile indicates that chelated iron (ferrous bis-glycine chelate) can work with ascorbic acid to achieve even higher absorption levels

- Separating intake of iron and inhibiting substances by a couple of hours.

- Using goats' milk instead of cows' milk.

- Gluten-free diet resolves some instances of iron-deficiency anemia, especially if the anemia is a result of celiac disease.

- It is believed[7][8] that "heme iron", found only in animal foods such as meat, fish and poultry, is more easily absorbed than "non-heme" iron, found in plant foods and supplements.

Iron bioavailability comparisons require stringent controls, because the largest factor affecting bioavailability is the subject's existing iron levels. Informal studies on bioavailability usually do not take this factor into account, so exaggerated claims from health supplement companies based on this sort of evidence should be ignored. Scientific studies are still in progress to determine which approaches yield the best results and the lowest costs.

If anemia does not respond to oral treatments, it may be necessary to administer iron parenterally (e.g., as iron dextran) using a drip or haemodialysis. Parenteral iron involves risks of fever, chills, backache, myalgia, dizziness, syncope, rash and anaphylactic shock. A follow up blood test is essential to demonstrate whether the treatment has been effective.

Iron supplements should be kept out of the reach of children, as iron-containing supplements are a frequent cause of poisoning in children.

Effect of Vitamin and Mineral Supplements

There is an observed correlation between serum retinol and hemoglobin levels. Women with a low serum retinol concentration are more likely to be iron-deficient and anemic, compared to those with normal to high levels of retinol. While vitamin A deficiency has an adverse effect on hemoglobin synthesis, even a slight increase in vitamin A intake can lead to a significant rise in hemoglobin levels. However, vitamin A is less effective in alleviating severe iron-deficiency anemia. Low levels of iron in the body cannot be relieved by vitamin A supplementation alone. Additionally, a low ascorbic acid stores in the body causes an impairment in the release of stored iron in the reticuloendothelial cells. Copper is necessary for iron uptake, and a copper deficiency can result in iron deficiency. Copper deficiency can sometimes be caused by excessive zinc or vitamin C supplementation.

I was diagnosed with anemia about 4–5 months ago. At that time I was taking a multi vitamin with iron. I then started SLow FE once a day for the 4–5 months. I have been having severe stomach pains, diarrhea, pains and just bloated and uncomfortable especially at night. I just got retested and my levels are now even lower since the last test. My gastrointestinal issues are getting worse. Any suggestions would be helpful?

You have been taking a very low dose (slow release) which is not a ~well absorbed~ type of iron to begin with. It has also been several months this has been happening so, yes, your iron levels could very well drop do to not enough iron intake. If this is a simple straight forward iron deficiency anemia due to heavy periods maybe then you probably just need a higher dose iron (guessing) that you can tolerate. Not all iron is created equally. I think but can't remember for sure and don't have time right now to research it, but I do believe that this is also an ~iron salts based~ iron which is very harsh and causes problems for many people. Then on the other hand some people cannot tolerate iron supplements at all and need IV iron infusions. I would suggest trying a different form of iron that is gastrointestinal friendly, higher dose, and that will work for you.

My gastroenterologist suggested to me to try Poly Iron 150 as an only resort. I feel that it saved my life because I was unable to tolerate iron at all. I could not even try IV iron due to my sensitivity.

SICKLE CELL ANEMIA

Sickle-cell disease, or sickle-cell anemia (or drepanocytosis), is a life-long blood disorder characterized by red blood cells that assume an abnormal, rigid, sickle shape. Sickling decreases the cells' flexibility and results in a risk of various complications. The sickling occurs because of a mutation in the hemoglobin gene. Life expectancy is shortened, with studies reporting an average life expectancy of 42 and 48 years for males and females, respectively.[1]

Sickle-cell disease, usually presenting in childhood, occurs more commonly in people (or their descendants) from parts of tropical and sub-tropical regions where malaria is or was common. One-third of all indigenous inhabitants of Sub-Saharan Africa carry the gene,[2] because in areas where malaria is common, there is a survival value in carrying only a single sickle-cell gene (sickle cell trait).[3] Those with only one of the two alleles of the sickle-cell disease are more resistant to malaria, since the infestation of the malaria plasmodium is halted by the sickling of the cells which it infests.

The prevalence of the disease in the United States is approximately 1 in 5,000, mostly affecting African

Americans, according to the National Institutes of Health.[4]

Classification

Sickle-cell anemia is the name of a specific form of sickle-cell disease in which there is homozygosity for the mutation that causes HbS. Sickle-cell anemia is also referred to as "HbSS", "SS disease", "haemoglobin S" or permutations thereof. In heterozygous people, who have only one sickle gene and one normal adult hemoglobin gene, it is referred to as "HbAS" or "sickle cell trait". Other, rarer forms of sickle-cell disease include sickle-haemoglobin C disease (HbSC), sickle beta-plus-thalassaemia (HbS/β^+) and sickle beta-zero-thalassaemia (HbS/β^0). These other forms of sickle-cell disease are compound heterozygous states in which the person has only one copy of the mutation that causes HbS and one copy of another abnormal haemoglobin allele.

The term *disease* is applied, because the inherited abnormality causes a pathological condition that can lead to death and severe complications. Not all inherited variants of haemoglobin are detrimental, a concept known as genetic polymorphism.

Sickle-cell anemia usually occurs in black children, but sometimes occurs in Hispanic children. About one in five hundred black children have it, and about one in 36,000 Hispanic children have sickle-cell anemia.[5]

Signs and Symptoms

Sickle-cell disease may lead to various acute and chronic complications, several of which are potentially lethal.

Vaso-Occlusive Crisis

The vaso-occlusive crisis is caused by sickle-shaped red blood cells that obstruct capillaries and restrict blood flow to an organ, resulting in ischemia, pain, and often organ damage. The frequency, severity, and duration of these crises vary considerably. Painful crises are treated with hydration and analgesics; pain management requires opioid administration at regular intervals until the crisis has settled. For milder crises, a subgroup of patients manage on NSAIDs (such as diclofenac or naproxen). For more severe crises, most patients require inpatient management for intravenous opioids; patient-controlled analgesia (PCA) devices are commonly used in this setting. Diphenhydramine is sometimes effective for the itching associated with the opioid use. Incentive spirometry, a technique to encourage deep breathing to minimise the development of atelectasis, is recommended.

Because of its narrow vessels and function in clearing defective red blood cells, the spleen is frequently affected. It is usually infarcted before the end of childhood in individuals suffering from sickle-cell anemia. This autosplenectomy increases the risk of infection from encapsulated organisms;[6][7] preventive antibiotics and vaccinations are recommended for those with such asplenia.

One of the earliest clinical manifestations is dactylitis, presenting as early as six months of age, and may occur in children with sickle trait.[8] The crisis can last up to a month.[9] Another recognised type of sickle crisis is the acute chest syndrome, a condition characterised by fever, chest pain, difficulty breathing, and pulmonary infiltrate on a chest X-ray. Given that pneumonia and sickling in the lung can both produce these symptoms, the patient is treated for both conditions. It can be triggered by painful crisis, respiratory infection, bone-marrow embolisation, or possibly by atelectasis, opiate administration, or surgery.

Most episodes of sickle cell crises last between five and seven days.[10]

Other Sickle-Cell Crises

• *Aplastic crises* are acute worsenings of the patient's baseline anemia, producing pallor, tachycardia, and fatigue. This crisis is triggered by parvovirus B19, which directly affects erythropoiesis (production of red blood cells). Parvovirus infection nearly completely prevents red blood cell production for two to three days. In normal individuals, this is of little consequence, but the shortened red cell life of sickle-cell patients results in an abrupt, life-threatening situation. Reticulocyte counts drop dramatically during the disease, and the rapid turnover of red cells leads to the drop in hemoglobin. Most patients can be managed supportively; some need blood transfusion.

• *Splenic sequestration crises* are acute, painful enlargements of the spleen. The abdomen becomes bloated and very hard. Management is supportive, sometimes with blood transfusion.

• *Hemolytic crises* are acute accelerated drops in hemoglobin level. The red blood cells break down at a faster rate. This is particularly common in patients with co-existent G6PD deficiency. Management is supportive, sometimes with blood transfusions.

Complications

Sickle-cell anemia can lead to various complications, including:

- Overwhelming post-(auto)splenectomy infection (OPSI), which is due to functional asplenia, caused by encapsulated organisms such as *Streptococcus pneumoniae* and *Haemophilus influenzae*. Daily penicillin prophylaxis is the most commonly used treatment during childhood, with some haematologists continuing treatment indefinitely. Patients benefit today from routine vaccination for *H. influenzae, S. pneumoniae,* and *Neisseria meningitidis.*

- Stroke, which can result from a progressive vascular narrowing of blood vessels, preventing oxygen from reaching the brain. Cerebral infarction occurs in children, and cerebral hemorrhage in adults.

- Cholelithiasis (gallstones) and cholecystitis, which may result from excessive bilirubin production and precipitation due to prolonged haemolysis.

- Jaundice, yellowing of the skin, may occur due to the inability of the liver to effectively remove bilirubin from the filtering of damaged red blood cells out of the blood supply as well as blocks in the organ's blood supply.[11][12]

- Avascular necrosis (aseptic bone necrosis) of the hip and other major joints, which may occur as a result of ischemia.

- Decreased immune reactions due to hyposplenism (malfunctioning of the spleen).

- Priapism and infarction of the penis.

- Osteomyelitis (bacterial bone infection), which is most frequently caused by *Salmonella* in individuals with sickle-cell disease, whereas *Staphylococcus* is the most common causative organism in the general population.

- Opioid tolerance, which can occur as a normal, physiologic response to the therapeutic use of opiates. Addiction to opiates occurs no more commonly among individuals with sickle-cell disease than among other individuals treated with opiates for other reasons.

- Acute papillary necrosis in the kidneys.

- Leg ulcers.

- In eyes, background retinopathy, proliferative retinopathy, vitreous hemorrhages and retinal detachments, resulting in blindness. Regular annual eye checks are recommended.

- During pregnancy, intrauterine growth retardation, spontaneous abortion, and pre-eclampsia.

- Chronic pain: Even in the absence of acute vaso-occlusive pain, many patients have chronic pain that is not reported[13].

- Pulmonary hypertension (increased pressure on the pulmonary artery), leading to strain on the right ventricle and a risk of heart failure; typical symptoms are shortness of breath, decreased exercise tolerance and episodes of syncope[14].

- Chronic renal failure—manifests itself with hypertension (high blood pressure), proteinuria (protein loss in the urine), hematuria (loss of red blood cells in urine) and worsened anemia. If it progresses to end-stage renal failure, it carries a poor prognosis.[15]

Heterozygotes

The heterozygous form (sickle cell trait) is almost always asymptomatic, and the only usual significant manifestation is the renal concentrating defect presenting with isosthenuria.

Diagnosis

In HbSS, the full blood count reveals haemoglobin levels in the range of 6–8 g/dL with a high reticulocyte count (as the bone marrow compensates for the destruction of sickle cells by producing more red blood cells). In other forms of sickle-cell disease, Hb levels tend to be higher. A blood film may show features of hyposplenism (target cells and Howell-Jolly bodies).

Sickling of the red blood cells, on a blood film, can be induced by the addition of sodium metabisulfite. The presence of sickle haemoglobin can also be demonstrated with the "sickle solubility test". A mixture of haemoglobin S (Hb S) in a reducing solution (such as sodium dithionite) gives a turbid appearance, whereas normal Hb gives a clear solution.

Abnormal haemoglobin forms can be detected on haemoglobin electrophoresis, a form of gel electrophoresis on which the various types of haemoglobin move at varying speeds. Sickle-cell haemoglobin (HgbS) and haemoglobin C with sickling (HgbSC)—the two most common forms—can be identified from there. The diagnosis can be confirmed with high-performance liquid chromatography

(HPLC). Genetic testing is rarely performed, as other investigations are highly specific for HbS and HbC.[16]

An acute sickle-cell crisis is often precipitated by infection. Therefore, a urinalysis to detect an occult UTI and CXR to look for occult pneumonia should be routinely performed.[17]

Pathophysiology

Sickle-cell anemia is caused by a point mutation in the β-globin chain of haemoglobin, causing the amino acid glutamic acid to be replaced with the hydrophobic amino acid valine at the sixth position. The β-globin gene is found on the short arm of chromosome 11. The association of two wild-type α -globin subunits with two mutant β-globin subunits forms haemoglobin S (HbS). Under low-oxygen conditions (being at high altitude, for example), the absence of a polar amino acid at position six of the β-globin chain promotes the non-covalent polymerisation (aggregation) of haemoglobin, which distorts red blood cells into a sickle shape and decreases their elasticity.

The loss of red blood cell elasticity is central to the pathophysiology of sickle-cell disease. Normal red blood cells are quite elastic, which allows the cells to deform to pass through capillaries. In sickle-cell disease, low-oxygen tension promotes red blood cell sickling and repeated episodes of sickling damage the cell membrane and decrease the cell's elasticity. These cells fail to return to normal shape when normal oxygen tension is restored. As a consequence, these rigid blood cells are unable to deform as they pass through narrow capillaries, leading to vessel occlusion and ischaemia.

The actual anemia of the illness is caused by hemolysis, the destruction of the red cells inside the spleen, because of their misshape. Although the bone marrow attempts to compensate by creating new red cells, it does not match the rate of destruction.[18] Healthy red blood cells typically live 90–120 days, but sickle cells only survive 10–20 days.[19]

Genetics

A single amino acid change causes haemoglobin proteins to form fibers.

Sickle-cell gene mutation probably arose spontaneously in different geographic areas, as suggested by restriction endonuclease analysis. These variants are known as Cameroon, Senegal, Benin, Bantu and Saudi-Asian. Their clinical importance springs from the fact that some of them are associated with higher HbF levels, e.g., Senegal and Saudi-Asian variants, and tend to have milder disease.[20]

In people heterozygous for HgbS (carriers of sickling haemoglobin), the polymerisation problems are minor, because the normal allele is able to produce over 50% of the haemoglobin. In people homozygous for HgbS, the presence of long-chain polymers of HbS distort the shape of the red blood cell from a smooth donut-like shape to ragged and full of spikes, making it fragile and susceptible to breaking within capillaries. Carriers have symptoms only if they are deprived of oxygen (for example, while climbing a mountain) or while severely dehydrated. Under normal circumstances, these painful crises occur 0.8 times per year per patient. The sickle-cell disease occurs when the seventh amino acid (if we count the initial methionine), glutamic acid, is replaced by valine to change its structure and function.

The gene defect is a known mutation of a single nucleotide (see single nucleotide polymorphism - SNP) (A to T) of the β-globin gene, which results in glutamate being substituted by valine at position 6. Haemoglobin S with this mutation are referred to as HbS, as opposed to the normal adult HbA. The genetic disorder is due to the mutation of a single nucleotide, from a GAG to GTG codon mutation. This is normally a benign mutation, causing *no* apparent effects on the secondary, tertiary, or quaternary structure of haemoglobin. What it does allow for, under conditions of low oxygen concentration, is the polymerization of the HbS itself. The deoxy form of haemoglobin exposes a hydrophobic patch on the protein between the E and F helices. The hydrophobic residues of the valine at position 6 of the beta chain in haemoglobin are able to associate with the hydrophobic patch, causing haemoglobin S molecules to aggregate and form fibrous precipitates.

The allele responsible for sickle-cell anemia is autosomal codominant and can be found on the short arm of chromosome 11. A person that receives the defective gene from both father and mother develops the disease; a person that receives one defective and one healthy allele remains healthy, but can pass on the disease and is known as a carrier. If two parents who are carriers have a child, there is a 1-in-4 chance of their child's developing the disease and a 1-in-2 chance of their child's being just a carrier. Since the gene is incompletely recessive, carriers can produce a few sickled red blood cells, not enough to cause symptoms, but enough to give resistance to malaria. Because of this, heterozygotes have a higher fitness than either of the homozygotes. This is known as heterozygote advantage.

Due to the adaptive advantage of the heterozygote, the disease is still prevalent, especially among people with recent ancestry in malaria-stricken areas, such as Africa, the Mediterranean, India and the Middle East.[21] Malaria was historically endemic to southern Europe, but it was declared eradicated in the mid-20th century, with the exception of rare sporadic cases.[22][23]

The Price equation is a simplified mathematical model of the genetic evolution of sickle-cell anemia.

The malaria parasite has a complex life cycle and spends part of it in red blood cells. In a carrier, the presence of the malaria parasite causes the red blood cells with defective haemoglobin to rupture prematurely, making the plasmodium unable to reproduce. Further, the polymerization of Hb affects the ability of the parasite to digest Hb in the first place. Therefore, in areas where malaria is a problem, people's chances of survival actually increase if they carry sickle-cell trait (selection for the heterozygote).

In the USA, where there is no endemic malaria, the prevalence of sickle-cell anemia among blacks is lower (about 0.25%) than in West Africa (about 4.0%)

and is falling. Without endemic malaria from Africa, the condition is purely disadvantageous and will tend to be bred out of the affected population. Another factor limiting the spread of sickle-cell genes in North America is the absence of cultural proclivities to polygamy.[24]

Sickle-cell disease is inherited in the autosomal recessive pattern.

Inheritance

• Sickle-cell conditions are inherited from parents in much the same way as blood type, hair color and texture, eye color, and other physical traits.

• The types of haemoglobin a person makes in the red blood cells depend upon what haemoglobin genes are inherited from his parents.

1. If one parent has sickle-cell anemia (SS) and the other has sickle-cell trait (AS), there is a 50% chance (or 1 out of 2) of a child's having sickle-cell disease (SS) and a 50% chance of a child's having sickle-cell trait (AS).

2. When both parents have sickle-cell trait (AS), they have a 25% chance (1 of 4) of a child's having sickle-cell disease (SS), as shown in the diagram.

Sickle-cell anemia appears to be caused by a codominant allele. Two carrier parents have a one in four chance of having a child with the disease (homozygous) and a one in two chance of having a child with an intermediate phenotype (heterozygous).[25]

Treatment

Dietary cyanate, from foods containing cyanide derivatives, has been used as a treatment for sickle- cell anemia.[26] In the laboratory, cyanate and thiocyanate irreversibly inhibit sickling of red blood cells drawn from sickle cell anemia patients.[27] However, the cyanate would have to be administered to the patient for a lifetime, as each new red blood cell created must be prevented from sickling at the time of creation. Cyanate also would be expelled via the urea of a patient every cycle of treatment.

Painful (Vaso-Occlusive) Crisis

Most people with sickle-cell disease have intensely painful episodes called vaso-occlusive crises. The frequency, severity, and duration of these crises, however, vary tremendously. Painful crises are treated symptomatically with analgesics; pain management requires opioid administration at regular intervals until the crisis has settled. For milder crises, a subgroup of patients manage on NSAIDs (such as diclofenac or naproxen). For more severe crises, most patients require inpatient management for intravenous opioids; patient-controlled analgesia (PCA) devices are commonly used in this setting. Diphenhydramine is also an effective agent that is frequently prescribed by doctors in order to help control any itching associated with the use of opioids.

Folic Acid and Penicillin

Children born with sickle-cell disease will undergo close observation by the pediatrician and will require management by a hematologist to assure they remain healthy. These patients will take a 1 mg dose of folic acid daily for life. From birth to five years of age, they will also have to take penicillin daily due to the immature immune system that makes them more prone to early childhood illnesses.

Acute Chest Crisis

Management is similar to vaso-occlusive crisis, with the addition of antibiotics (usually a quinolone or macrolide, since wall-deficient ["atypical"] bacteria are thought to contribute to the syndrome),[28] oxygen supplementation for hypoxia, and close observation.

Should the pulmonary infiltrate worsen or the oxygen requirements increase, simple blood transfusion or exchange transfusion is indicated. The latter involves the exchange of a significant portion of the patients red cell mass for normal red cells, which decreases the percent of haemoglobin S in the patient's blood.

Hydroxyurea

The first approved drug for the causative treatment of sickle-cell anemia, hydroxyurea, was shown to decrease the number and severity of attacks in a study in 1995 (Charache *et al.*)[29] and shown to possibly increase survival time in a study in 2003 (Steinberg *et al.*).[30] This is achieved, in part, by reactivating fetal haemoglobin production in place of the haemoglobin S that causes sickle-cell anemia. Hydroxyurea had previously been used as a chemotherapy agent, and there is some concern that long-term use may be harmful, but this risk has been shown to be either absent or very small and it is likely that the benefits outweigh the risks.[31]

Bone Marrow Transplants

Bone marrow transplants have proven to be effective in children.[32]

Future Treatments

Various approaches are being sought for preventing sickling episodes as well as for the complications of sickle-cell disease. Other ways to modify hemoglobin switching are being investigated, including the use of phytochemicals such as nicosan. Gene therapy is under investigation.

Another treatment being investigated is Senicapoc.

Situation of Carriers

People who are known carriers of the disease often undergo genetic counseling before they have a child. A test to see if an unborn child has the disease takes either a blood sample from the fetus or a sample of amniotic fluid. Since taking a blood sample from a fetus has greater risks, the latter test is usually used.

After the mutation responsible for this disease was discovered in 1979, the U.S. Air Force required black applicants to test for the mutation. It dismissed 143 applicants because they were carriers, even though none of them had the condition. It eventually withdrew the requirement, but only after a trainee filed a lawsuit.[33]

History

This collection of clinical findings was unknown until the explanation of the sickle cells in 1904 by the Chicago cardiologist and professor of medicine James B. Herrick (1861–1954), whose intern Ernest Edward Irons (1877–1959) found "peculiar elongated and sickle-shaped" cells in the blood of Walter Clement Noel, a 20-year-old first-year dental student from Grenada, after Noel was admitted to the Chicago Presbyterian Hospital in December 1904 suffering from anemia.[34]

Noel was readmitted several times over the next three years for "muscular rheumatism" and "bilious attacks". Noel completed his studies and returned to the capital of Grenada (St. George's) to practice dentistry. He died of pneumonia in 1916 and is buried in the Catholic cemetery at Sauteurs in the north of Grenada.[35]

The disease was named "sickle-cell anemia" by Vernon Mason in 1922. However, some elements of the disease had been recognized earlier: A paper in the *Southern Journal of Medical Pharmacology* in 1846 described the absence of a spleen in the autopsy of a runaway slave. The African medical literature reported this condition in the 1870s, when it was known locally as *ogbanjes* ("children who come and go") because of the very high infant mortality rate caused by this condition. A history of the condition tracked reports back to 1670 in one Ghanaian family.[36] Also, the practice of using tar soap to cover blemishes caused by sickle-cell sores was prevalent in the black community.

Linus Pauling and colleagues were the first, in 1949, to demonstrate that sickle-cell disease occurs as a result of an abnormality in the haemoglobin molecule. This was the first time a genetic disease was linked to a mutation of a specific protein, a milestone in the history of molecular biology, and it was published in their paper "Sickle Cell Anemia, a Molecular Disease".

The origin of the mutation that led to the sickle-cell gene was initially thought to be in the Arabian peninsula, spreading to Asia and Africa. It is now known, from evaluation of chromosome structures, that there have been at least four independent mutational events, three in Africa and a fourth in either Saudi Arabia or central India. These independent events occurred between 3,000 and 6,000 generations ago, approximately 70–150,000 years.

HEMOLYTIC ANEMIA

Hemolytic anemia is anemia due to hemolysis, the abnormal breakdown of red blood cells (RBCs) either in the blood vessels (intravascular hemolysis) or elsewhere in the body (extravascular). It has numerous possible causes, ranging from relatively harmless to life-threatening. The general classification of hemolytic anemia is either acquired or inherited. Treatment depends on the cause and nature of the breakdown.

In a healthy person, a red blood cell survives 90 to 120 days (on average) in the circulation, so about 1% of human red blood cells break down each day. The spleen (part of the reticulo-endothelial system) is the main organ which removes old and damaged RBCs from the circulation. In healthy individuals, the break down and removal of RBCs from the circulation is matched by the production of new RBCs in the bone marrow.

In conditions where the rate of RBC breakdown is increased, the body initially compensates by producing more RBCs; however, breakdown of RBCs can exceed the rate that the body can make RBCs, and so anemia can develop. Bilirubin, a breakdown product of hemoglobin, can accumulate in the blood causing jaundice, and be excreted in the urine causing the urine to become a dark brown colour.

Symptoms

Signs of anemia (fatigue and, later, heart failure) are generally present. Jaundice may be present. Certain aspects of the medical history can suggest a cause for hemolysis, such as drugs, fava bean or other sensitivity, prosthetic heart valve, or another medical illness.

Tests

• Peripheral blood smear microscopy:

  • fragments of the red blood cells ("schistocytes") can be present

  • some red blood cells may appear smaller and rounder than usual (spherocytes)

  • Reticulocytes are present in elevated numbers. This may be overlooked if a special stain is not used.

• The level of unconjugated bilirubin in the blood is elevated. This may lead to jaundice.

• The level of lactate dehydrogenase (LDH) in the blood is elevated

- Haptoglobin levels are decreased

- If the direct Coombs test is positive, hemolysis is caused by an immune process.

- Haemosiderin in the urine indicates chronic intravascular haemolysis. There is also urobilinogen in the urine.

Clinical findings in haemolytic anemias:

- increased serum bilirubin levels in blood, therefore jaundice

- pallor in mucous membrane and skin

- increased urobilinogen in urine

- Splenomegaly

- Pigmented gallstones may be found.

My mom is 80 and was just diagnosed with hemolytic anemia. She was put on a high dose of prednisone and her RBC is starting to come back to normal. It has taken about 10 days. She has lost a couple of pounds and is very tired. She has been healthy all of her life and then went in for a cholesterol check and this showed up in her blood work. Very strange. The doctor has not said anything about any underlying illness...

*should we be concerned about that? I think
because she is responding to the prednisone he
is pleased with that. I am hearing and reading
so many bad things about prednisone, but it
seems like if it is short term it can't do too much
damage. I am sure it has saved many lives.
Does anyone have anything good to say about
prednisone? Any helpful information for my mom
would be appreciated.*

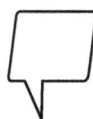

*I was on prednisone the first year I was diagnosed,
they should give you between 30mg and 60mg if
you don't respond they increase it. I didn't respond
so I was on 120mg for quite a while once your
levels start remounting… everyone is different, they
start tapering it 10mg at a time. The side effects
are what they are, swelling also called Cushings
Syndrome, anxiety, hunger, insomnia. You have
to bear with it; it saved my life amongst other
treatments. Doing mild exercise helps, I suppose at
80 it can be difficult.*

*Hemolytic anemia seems to be diagnosed when
other things go wrong by what I've experienced
and heard by other sufferers, in my case I
had virus like symptoms and developed into
pneumonia. They don't keep you on prednisone
permanently as the side effects… loss of calcium*

in the bones mainly they might taper her off it and get her on azatriopin, an immunosuppressant.

Also they should give her folic acid. Folic acid helps the bone marrow while producing blood. As Hemolysis is the destruction of blood your bone marrow needs to work extra hard to make new blood and folic acid helps it not to suffer!

Is your mom seeing a hematologist? The doctor would do testing to see if there is an underlying cause. My husband was diagnosed a few years ago. He was on prednisone but it didn't control it too well and increases made him feel really bad. He ended up having his spleen removed at which time the surgeon did a bone marrow biopsy, liver biopsy and checked around to see any cancer. He was clear. He retired from his job, not because of the anemia, it was planned and we switched to a different health insurance. The new hematologist thought maybe removing the spleen was a bit premature and would have tried different drugs first. He is in remission now, his blood tests are wacky but his blood cells aren't being destroyed prematurely. He take folic acid and is monitored every few months. He has to be very careful about being exposed to illness as not having a spleen can dangerously affect him should he get sick.

However, he is back on the golf course and feeling so much better.

Is it unusual to have darker patches of skin on some areas of your body?

I have this - on my right forearm. It is quite recent. It has gradually grown to involve a larger area, all the way to my wrist. I'd describe it as a series of interlocking lines with a few solid spots here and there.

Hyperpigmentation is normally caused by melanin, a pigment. Melanin is produced by cells called melanocytes, located in the skin.

I just read that sometimes the darkening of the skin may be due to an iron pigment left behind when the red blood cells die.

I have it on my forehead. I just got it within the last few years (when my iron was low), but not sure if it has anything to do with it. I thought it was more my adrenal issues...

Classification of Hemolytic Anemias

Causes of hemolytic anemia can be either genetic or acquired.

Genetic

Genetic causes can involve the RBC membrane, metabolism, or hemoglobin conditions.

Acquired

Acquired hemolytic anemia can be divided into immune and non-immune mediated.

Differential Diagnosis

- Ineffective hematopoiesis is sometimes misdiagnosed as hemolysis.

  - Clinically these conditions may share many features of hemolysis

  - Red cell breakdown occurs before a fully developed red cell is released into the circulation.

  - Examples: thalassemia, myelodysplastic syndrome

- Megaloblastic anemia due to deficiency in vitamin B-12 or folic acid.

Therapy

Definitive therapy depends on the cause.

- Symptomatic treatment can be given by blood transfusion, if there is marked anemia.

- In severe immune-related hemolytic anemia, steroid therapy is sometimes necessary.

- Sometimes splenectomy can be helpful where extravascular hemolysis is predominant (i.e. most of the red blood cells are being removed by the spleen).

HEMOGLOBIN

Hemoglobin (also abbreviated as Hb or Hgb) is the iron-containing oxygen-transport metalloprotein in the red blood cells of vertebrates,[1] and the tissues of some invertebrates.

In mammals, the protein makes up about 97% of the red blood cell's dry content, and around 35% of the total content (including water). Hemoglobin transports oxygen from the lungs or gills to the rest of the body where it releases the oxygen for cell use. It also has a variety of other roles of gas transport and effect-modulation which vary from species to species, and are quite diverse in some invertebrates.

Hemoglobin has an oxygen binding capacity of between 1.36 and 1.37 ml O_2 per gram Hemoglobin,[2] which increases the total blood oxygen capacity seventyfold.[3]

I am exhausted and weak and getting worse. My Hemoglobin is 9.1. I'm taking iron, have had an endoscopy and colonoscopy and am scheduled for a capsule endoscopy. So far all that was found was a bleeding hemorrhoid.

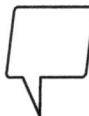

A person can have low iron levels for one or more of three reasons:

Blood loss, either from having a disease or injury, not getting enough iron in the daily diet such as vegetarians and/or not being able to absorb the iron in the diet as seen in malabsorption syndromes.

It is unlikely that your bleeding hemorrhoid caused this low of a number unless it is a severe grade and have more than one. It does happen though if it is bad.

The small intestines are many times where you will find answers and many times this test is overlooked too so it's great that your doc is moving forward for you. I have heard that less than 5% of bleeds occur in the small intestines. Being a male, it's a little different when anemic because they already know that you don't have a regular monthly cycle. For women they just blame that and often times it's something else as a cause which is found at a later date so in that regard you're a step above the rest for finding a cause.

You are considered moderately anemic; although you are feeling poorly you have time to find a cause without stressing too much. I wonder what your ferritin and iron panel look like. The CBC tells if you are anemic which we know you are already. The iron tests tell how much of the iron in the body is available and how much has been used up. There can also be an elevated ferritin in the presence of some autoimmune conditions which is a possibility for you. When I was anemic I was very ill with many strange things happening so I didn't wait too long for someone to help me I made appointments with the Hematologist (unable to take iron and levels continued to drop) next I saw a Rheumatologist to rule out AI causes (which were 3 pages full) and finally, a Neurologist as well.

Have you also had your B-12 and folate checked? It should be. IF intrinsic factor in the stomach and Celiac disease are the major ones to check for and even H-Pylori bacteria although you have no ulcers. All simple blood tests, not so simple to get the doctor to check at times.

I got my lab results back for suspected anemia. My hemoglobin was 14, he is retesting for ferritin levels because I had been supplementing iron at the time of the test. But my TSH level was 8, but T3 and T4 normal. For anyone with thyroid disease, does this mean I am hypothyroid? And could the ferritin levels below with a hemoglobin of 14, and are anemia and hypothyroid somehow related?

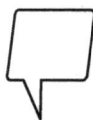

I got my lab results back for suspected anemia. My hemoglobin was 14, he is retesting for ferritin levels because I had been supplementing iron at the time of the test.

14 is optimal. I will give you an example of what you are asking. After my anemia 8.5 hgb, and coming up from 2 ferritin, my Hgb finally hit 14.4 and I had a 41 Ferritin at that time. This however will be different for everyone. You have to have some stores to have such a high Hgb. Now/ low ferritin is the end stage of the ferritin stores resulting in anemia. In the future, you should never begin iron supplements until you know all your numbers and a cause to support that. Anemia has many symptoms that mimic many other things, one of them commonly being thyroid.

Degradation in Vertebrate Animals

When red cells reach the end of their life due to aging or defects, they are broken down, the hemoglobin molecule is broken up and the iron gets recycled. When the porphyrin ring is broken up, the fragments are normally secreted in the bile by the liver. This process also produces one molecule of carbon monoxide for every molecule of heme degraded.[25] This is one of the few natural sources of carbon monoxide production in the human body, and is responsible for the normal blood levels of carbon monoxide even in people breathing pure air. The other major final product of heme degradation is bilirubin. Increased levels of this chemical are detected in the blood if red cells are being destroyed more rapidly than usual. Improperly degraded hemoglobin protein or hemoglobin that has been released from the blood cells too rapidly can clog small blood vessels, especially the delicate blood filtering vessels of the kidneys, causing kidney damage.

Role in Disease

In sickle cell hemoglobin (HbS) glutamic acid in position 6 (in beta chain) is mutated to valine. This change allows the deoxygenated form of the hemoglobin to stick to each other.

Hemoglobin deficiency can be caused either by decrease amount of hemoglobin molecules as in anemia, or decreased ability of each molecule to bind oxygen at the same partial pressure of oxygen. hemoglobinopathies (genetic defects resulting in abnormal structure of the hemoglobin molecule[26]) may cause both. In any case, hemoglobin deficiency decreases blood oxygen-carrying capacity. Hemoglobin deficiency is generally strictly distinguished from hypoxemia, defined as decreased partial pressure of oxygen in blood,[27][28][29][30] although both are causes of hypoxia (insufficient oxygen supply to tissues).

The ability of each hemoglobin molecule to carry oxygen is normally modified by altered blood pH or CO_2, causing an altered oxygen-haemoglobin dissociation curve. However, it can also be pathologically altered in e.g. carbon monoxide poisoning.

Decrease of hemoglobin, with or without an absolute decrease of red blood cells, leads to symptoms of anemia. Anemia has many different causes, although iron deficiency and its resultant iron deficiency anemia are the most common causes in the Western world. As absence of iron decreases heme synthesis, red blood cells in iron deficiency anemia are *hypochromic* (lacking the red hemoglobin pigment) and *microcytic* (smaller than normal). Other anemias are rarer. In hemolysis (accelerated breakdown of red blood cells), associated jaundice is caused by the hemoglobin metabolite bilirubin, and the circulating hemoglobin can cause renal failure.

Some mutations in the globin chain are associated with the hemoglobinopathies, such as sickle-cell disease and thalassemia. Other mutations, as discussed at the beginning of the article, are benign and are referred to merely as hemoglobin variants.

There is a group of genetic disorders, known as the *porphyrias* that are characterized by errors in metabolic pathways of heme synthesis. King George III of the United Kingdom was probably the most famous porphyria sufferer.

To a small extent, hemoglobin A slowly combines with glucose at the terminal valine (an alpha aminoacid) of each β chain. The resulting molecule is often referred to as Hb A_{1c}. As the concentration of glucose in the blood increases, the percentage of Hb A that turns into Hb A_{1c} increases. In diabetics whose glucose usually runs high, the percent Hb A_{1c} also runs high. Because of the slow rate of Hb A combination with glucose, the Hb A_{1c} percentage is representative of glucose level in the blood averaged over a longer time (the half-life of red blood cells, which is typically 50–55 days).

Elevated levels of hemoglobin are associated with increased numbers or sizes of red blood cells, called polycythemia. This elevation may be caused by congenital heart disease, cor pulmonale, pulmonary fibrosis, too much erythropoietin, or polycythemia vera.[31]

Diagnostic Uses

Hemoglobin concentration measurement is among the most commonly performed blood tests, usually as part of a complete blood count. For example it is typically tested before blood donation. Results are reported in g/L, g/dL or mol/L. 1 g/dL equals about 0.6206 mmol/L. Normal levels are:

Men: 13.5 to 16.5 g/dl

Women: 12.1 to 15.1 g/dl

Children: 11 to 16 g/dl

Pregnant women: 11 to 12 g/dl[32]

Normal values of hemoglobin in 1st and 3rd trimester of pregnant women must be at least 11 g/dl and at least 10.5 g/dl during 2nd trimester.[33]

If the concentration is below normal, this is called anemia. Anemias are classified by the size of red blood cells, the cells which contain hemoglobin in vertebrates. The anemia is called "microcytic" if red cells are small, "macrocytic" if they are large, and "normocytic" otherwise.

Hematocrit, the proportion of blood volume occupied by red blood cells, is typically about three times the hemoglobin level. For example, if the hemoglobin is measured at 17, that compares with a hematocrit of 51.[34]

Long-term control of blood sugar concentration can be measured by the concentration of Hb A_{1c}. Measuring it directly would require many samples because blood sugar levels vary widely through the day. Hb A_{1c} is the product of the irreversible reaction of hemoglobin A with glucose. A higher glucose concentration results in more Hb A_{1c}. Because the reaction is slow, the Hb A_{1c} proportion represents glucose level in blood averaged over the half-life of red blood cells, is typically 50–55 days. An Hb A_{1c} proportion of 6.0% or less show good long-term glucose control, while values above 7.0% are elevated. This test is especially useful for diabetics.[35]

The functional magnetic resonance imaging (fMRI) machine may use the signal from oxyhemoglobin as it partially aligns these molecules with the magnetic field. The machine sends a series of magnetic pulses at the participant's head or other body structure, slowly knocking the molecules out of alignment, and a radio wave is emitted when they are back in alignment. The machine can then pick up these signals and use them to make scans, which are cross-sectional maps showing blood flow.

REFERENCES – ANEMIA

1. MedicineNet.com --> Definition of Anemia Last Editorial Review: 12/9/2000 8:31:00 AM

2. merriam-webster dictionary --> anemia Retrieved on May 25, 2009

3. eMedicine - Anemia, Chronic : Article by Fredrick M Abrahamian, DO, FACEP

4. answers.com - The American Heritage Dictionary of the English Language, Fourth Edition --> Anemia Retrieved on May 25, 2009

5. britannica.com --> blood disease, stating hypoxemia (reduced oxygen tension in the blood). Retrieved on May 25, 2009

6. Biology-Online.org --> Dictionary » H » Hypoxemia last modified 00:05, 29 December 2008

7. Page 430 -> Pathophysiology of acute respiratory failure in Trauma By William C. Wilson, Christopher M. Grande, David B. Hoyt Edition: illustrated Published by CRC Press, 2007 ISBN 082472920X, 9780824729202 1384 pages

8. Hazards of hypoxemia: How to protect your patient from low oxygen levels In Nursing , May 1996 by McGaffigan, Patricia A

9. eMedicineHealth > anemia article Author: Saimak T. Nabili, MD, MPH. Editor: Melissa Conrad Stöppler, MD. Last Editorial Review: 12/9/2008. Retrieved on 4 April, 2009

10. World Health Organization (2008). Worldwide prevalence of anemia 1993-2005. Geneva: World Health Organization. ISBN 9789241596657. http://whqlibdoc. who.int/publications/2008/9789241596657_eng.pdf. Retrieved on 2009-03-25.

11. Recommendations to Prevent and Control Iron Deficiency in the United States MMWR 1998;47 (No. RR-3) p. 5

12. Iron Deficiency Anaemia: Assessment, Prevention, and Control: A guide for programme managers

13. eMedicine - Vitamin B-12 Associated Neurological Diseases : Article by Niranjan N Singh, MD, DM, DNB July 18, 2006

14. Physiology or Medicine 1934 - Presentation Speech

15. Dorlands Medical Dictionary

16. Onions are Toxic to Cats

17. Hébert PC, Wells G, Blajchman MA, et al. (1999). "A multicenter, randomized, controlled clinical trial of transfusion requirements in critical care. Transfusion Requirements in Critical Care Investigators, Canadian Critical Care Trials Group". N. Engl. J. Med. 340 (6): 409–17. PMID 9971864.

18. Bush RL, Pevec WC, Holcroft JW (1997). "A prospective, randomized trial limiting perioperative red blood cell transfusions in vascular patients". *Am. J. Surg.* **174** (2): 143–8. doi:10.1016/S0002-9610(97)00073-1. PMID 9293831.

19. Bracey AW, Radovancevic R, Riggs SA, et al. (1999). "Lowering the hemoglobin threshold for transfusion in coronary artery bypass procedures: effect on patient outcome". *Transfusion* **39** (10): 1070–7. doi:10.1046/j.1537-2995.1999.39101070.x. PMID 10532600.

20. McIntyre LA, Fergusson DA, Hutchison JS, et al. (2006). "Effect of a liberal versus restrictive transfusion strategy on mortality in patients with moderate to severe head injury". *Neurocritical care* **5** (1): 4–9. doi:10.1385/NCC:5:1:4. PMID 16960287.

21. Corwin HL, Gettinger A, Pearl RG, et al. (2004). "The CRIT Study: Anemia and blood transfusion in the critically ill--current clinical practice in the United States". *Crit. Care Med.* **32** (1): 39–52. doi:10.1097/01.CCM.0000104112.34142.79. PMID 14707558.

22. Vincent JL, Baron JF, Reinhart K, et al. (2002). "Anemia and blood transfusion in critically ill patients". *JAMA* **288** (12): 1499–507. doi:10.1001/jama.288.12.1499. PMID 12243637.

23. Undersea and Hyperbaric Medical Society. "Exceptional Blood Loss - Anemia". http://www.uhms.org/ResourceLibrary/Indications/ExceptionalBloodLossAnemia/tabid/277/Default.aspx. Retrieved on 2008-05-19.

24. Hart GB, Lennon PA, Strauss MB. (1987). "Hyperbaric oxygen in exceptional acute blood-loss anemia". *J. Hyperbaric Med* **2** (4): 205–210. http://archive.rubicon-foundation.org/4352. Retrieved on 2008-05-19.

25. Van Meter KW (2005). "A systematic review of the application of hyperbaric oxygen in the treatment of severe anemia: an evidence-based approach". *Undersea Hyperb Med* 32 (1): 61–83. PMID 15796315. http://archive.rubicon-foundation.org/4038. Retrieved on 2008-05-19.

REFERENCES – MEGALOBLASTIC ANEMIA

1. "Megaloblastic Anemia: Overview - eMedicine Hematology". http://emedicine. medscape.com/article/204066-overview. Retrieved on 2009-02-07.

2. "Megaloblastic (Pernicious) Anemia - Lucile Packard Children's Hospital". http://www.lpch.org/DiseaseHealthInfo/HealthLibrary/hematology/megalob. html. Retrieved on 2008-03-12.

3. Savage DG, Lindenbaum J, Stabler SP, Allen RH (1994). "Sensitivity of serum methylmalonic acid and total homocysteine determinations for diagnosing cobalamin and folate deficiencies". *Am. J. Med.* **96** (3): 239–46. doi:10.1016/0002-9343(94)90149-X. PMID 8154512. http://linkinghub.elsevier. com/retrieve/pii/0002-9343(94)90149-X.

REFERENCES – IRON DEFICIENCY ANEMIA

1. Brady PG (2007). "Iron deficiency anemia: a call for aggressive diagnostic evaluation". *South. Med. J.* **100** (10): 966–7. doi:10.1097/SMJ.0b013e3181520699. PMID 17943034. http://meta.wkhealth.com/pt/pt-core/template-journal/lwwgateway/media/landingpage.htm?doi=10.1097/SMJ.0b013e3181520699.

2. Calis JC, Phiri KS, Faragher EB, *et al.* (2008). "Severe anemia in Malawian children". *N. Engl. J. Med.* **358** (9): 888–99. doi:10.1056/NEJMoa072727. PMID 18305266. http://content.nejm.org/cgi/pmidlookup?view=short&pmid=18305 266&promo=ONFLNS19.

3. Dreyfuss ML, Stoltzfus RJ, Shrestha JB, *et al.* (2000). "Hookworms, malaria and vitamin A deficiency contribute to anemia and iron deficiency among pregnant women in the plains of Nepal". *J. Nutr.* **130** (10): 2527–36. PMID 11015485.

4. Mazza, J.; Barr, R. M.; McDonald, J. W.; and Valberg, L. S.; (21 Oct 1978). "Usefulness of the serum ferritin concentration in the detection of iron deficiency in a general hospital". *Canadian Medical Association Journal* **119** (8): 884–886. PMID 737638. http://www.cmaj.ca/cgi/content/abstract/119/8/884. Retrieved on 2009-05-04.

5. Kis, AM; Carnes, M (July 1998). "Detecting iron deficiency in anemic patients with concomitant medical problems.". *J Gen Intern Med.* **13** (7): 455–61. doi:10.1046/j.1525-1497.1998.00134.x. PMID 9686711.

6. Thomason, Ronald W.; Almiski, Muhamad S. (April 2009). "Evidence That Stainable Bone Marrow Iron Following Parenteral Iron Therapy Does Not Correlate With Serum Iron Studies and May Not Represent Readily Available Storage Iron". *American Journal of Clinical Pathology* **131**: 580–585. doi:10.1309/AJCPBAY9KRZF8NUC. PMID 19289594. http://ajcp.ascpjournals.org/content/131/4/580.full. Retrieved on 2009-05-04.

7. Health Canada. "Dietary Sources of Iron". Government of Canada. http://www.hc-sc.gc.ca/fn-an/nutrition/prenatal/national_guidelines-lignes_directrices_nationales-07-table2-eng.php. Retrieved on 2009-03-30.

8. National Institutes of Health. "Dietary Supplement Fact Sheet: Iron". United States of America, Department of Health and Human Services. http://ods.od.nih.gov/factsheets/iron.asp. Retrieved on 2009-03-30.

REFERENCES – SICKLE CELL ANEMIA

1. Platt OS, Brambilla DJ, Rosse WF, *et al.* (June 1994). "Mortality in sickle cell disease. Life expectancy and risk factors for early death". *N. Engl. J. Med.* **330** (23): 1639–44. doi:10.1056/NEJM199406093302303. PMID 7993409. http://content.nejm.org/cgi/content/full/330/23/1639.

2. Sicklecell.md

3. Sicklecell.md FAQ: "Why is Sickle Cell Anaemia only found in Black people?

4. http://www.nhlbi.nih.gov/health/dci/Diseases/Sca/SCA_Summary.html

5. http://www.nhlbi.nih.gov/health/dci/Diseases/Sca/SCA_WhoIsAtRisk.html

6. Pearson H. "Sickle cell anemia and severe infections due to encapsulated bacteria". *J Infect Dis* **136** Suppl: S25–30. PMID 330779.

7. Wong W, Powars D, Chan L, Hiti A, Johnson C, Overturf G (1992). "Polysaccharide encapsulated bacterial infection in sickle cell anemia: a thirty year epidemiologic experience". *Am J Hematol* **39** (3): 176–82. doi:10.1002/ajh.2830390305. PMID 1546714.

8. http://www.pubmedcentral.nih.gov/articlerender.fcgi?artid=1345873

9. http://www.ejbjs.org/cgi/content/abstract/58/8/1161

10. "BestBets: How long should an average sickle cell crisis last?". http://www.bestbets.org/bets/bet.php?id=1189.

11. "Sickle cell anemia". Mayo Clinic. 2009-04-01. http://www.mayoclinic.com/health/sickle-cell-anemia/DS00324/DSECTION=symptoms. Retrieved on 2009-05-02.

12. Bandyopadhyay R, Bandyopadhyay SK, Dutta A (2008). "Sickle cell hepatopathy". *Indian J Pathol Microbiol* **51** (2): 284–5. doi:10.4103/0377-4929.41698. PMID 18603711. http://www.ijpmonline.org/article.asp?issn=0377-4929;year=2008;volume=51;issue=2;spage=284;epage=285;aulast=Bandyopadhyay.

13. Smith WR, Penberthy LT, Bovbjerg VE, *et al.* (2008). "Daily assessment of pain in adults with sickle cell disease". *Ann. Intern. Med.* **148** (2): 94–101. PMID 18195334.

14. Gladwin MT, Sachdev V, Jison ML, *et al.* (2004). "Pulmonary hypertension as a risk factor for death in patients with sickle cell disease". *N. Engl. J. Med.* **350** (9): 886–95. doi:10.1056/NEJMoa035477. PMID 14985486. http://content.nejm.org/cgi/content/full/350/9/886.

15. Powars DR, Elliott-Mills DD, Chan L, *et al.* (1991). "Chronic renal failure in sickle cell disease: risk factors, clinical course, and mortality". *Ann. Intern. Med.* **115** (8): 614–20. PMID 1892333.

16. Clarke GM, Higgins TN (2000). "Laboratory investigation of hemoglobinopathies and thalassemias: review and update". *Clin. Chem.* **46** (8 Pt 2): 1284–90. PMID 10926923. http://www.clinchem.org/cgi/content/full/46/8/1284.

17. "BestBets: Does routine urinalysis and chest radiography detect occult bacterial infection in sickle cell patients presenting to the accident and emergency department with painful crisis?". http://www.bestbets.org/bets/bet.php?id=1102.

18. http://sickle.bwh.harvard.edu/scd_background.html

19. http://emedicine.medscape.com/article/778971-overview

20. Green NS, Fabry ME, Kaptue-Noche L, Nagel RL (1993). "Senegal haplotype is associated with higher HbF than Benin and Cameroon haplotypes in African children with sickle cell anemia". *Am. J. Hematol.* **44** (2): 145–6. doi:10.1002/ajh.2830440214. PMID 7505527.

21. Kwiatkowski DP (2005). "How malaria has affected the human genome and what human genetics can teach us about malaria". *Am. J. Hum. Genet.* **77** (2): 171–92. doi:10.1086/432519. PMID 16001361. Full text at PMC: 1224522

22. http://www.cdc.gov/ncidod/EID/vol7no6/romi.htm

23. http://www.pubmedcentral.nih.gov/articlerender.fcgi?artid=1808464

24. http://journals.cambridge.org/action/displayAbstract?aid=1361276

25. "The Open Door Web Site : IB Biology : Genetics : Co-dominance." The Open Door Web Site : Home Page. 9 Sep. 2007. 30 Dec. 2008 <http://www.saburchill.com/IBbiology/chapters03/004.html>

26. http://www.clarafelixclinic.org/assets/further_info/cyanate_houston.pdf

27. http://www.clarafelixclinic.org/assets/further_info/thiocyanate_agbai.pdf

28. Aldrich TK, Nagel RL. (1998). "Pulmonary Complications of Sickle Cell Disease.". in C et al., editors. *Pulmonary and Critical Care Medicine* (6th ed.). St. Louis: Mosby. pp. pp.1–10. ISBN 0-81511-371-4.

29. Charache S, Terrin ML, Moore RD, et al. (1995). "Effect of hydroxyurea on the frequency of painful crises in sickle cell anemia. Investigators of the Multicenter Study of Hydroxyurea in Sickle Cell Anemia". *N. Engl. J. Med.* **332** (20): 1317–22. doi:10.1056/NEJM199505183322001. PMID 7715639.

30. Steinberg MH, Barton F, Castro O, et al. (2003). "Effect of hydroxyurea on mortality and morbidity in adult sickle cell anemia: risks and benefits up to 9 years of treatment". *JAMA* **289** (13): 1645–51. doi:10.1001/jama.289.13.1645. PMID 12672732. http://jama.ama-assn.org/cgi/content/full/289/13/1645.

31. Platt OS (2008). "Hydroxyurea for the treatment of sickle cell anemia". *N. Engl. J. Med.* **358** (13): 1362–9. doi:10.1056/NEJMct0708272. PMID 18367739.

32. Walters MC, Patience M, Leisenring W, *et al.* (August 1996). "Bone marrow transplantation for sickle cell disease". *N. Engl. J. Med.* **335** (6): 369–76. doi:10.1056/NEJM199608083350601. PMID 8663884. http://content.nejm.org/cgi/pmidlookup?view=short&pmid=8663884&promo=ONFLNS19.

33. Anonymous (4 January 1981). "Air force academy sued over sickle cell policy". *New York Times.* http://query.nytimes.com/gst/fullpage.html?sec=health&res=9807EFD7163BF937A35752C0A967948260. Retrieved on 21 December 2008.

34. {author=Herrick, J.B. |title=Peculiar elongated and sickle-shaped red blood corpuscles in a case of severe anemia |journal=Archives of Internal Medicine |volume=6 | pages=517-521 |year=1910

35. Savitt TL, Goldberg MF (1989). "Herrick's 1910 case report of sickle cell anemia. The rest of the story". *JAMA* **261** (2): 266–71. doi:10.1001/jama.261.2.266. PMID 2642320.

36. Konotey-Ahulu FID. Effect of environment on sickle cell disease in West Africa: epidemiologic and clinical considerations. In: Sickle Cell Disease, Diagnosis, Management, Education and Research. Abramson H, Bertles JF, Wethers DL, eds. CV Mosby Co, St. Louis. 1973; 20; cited in Desai, D. V.; Hiren Dhanani (2004). "Sickle Cell Disease: History And Origin". *The Internet Journal of Haematology* **1** (2). ISSN 1540-2649. http://www.ispub.com/ostia/index.php?xmlFilePath=journals/ijhe/vol1n2/sickle.xml.

37. Desai, D. V.; Hiren Dhanani (2004). "Sickle Cell Disease: History And Origin". *The Internet Journal of Haematology* **1** (2). ISSN 1540-2649. http://www.ispub.com/ostia/index.php?xmlFilePath=journals/ijhe/vol1n2/sickle.xml.

REFERENCES – HEMOGLOBIN

1. Maton, Anthea; Jean Hopkins, Charles William McLaughlin, Susan Johnson, Maryanna Quon Warner, David LaHart, Jill D. Wright (1993). *Human Biology and Health.* Englewood Cliffs, New Jersey, USA: Prentice Hall. ISBN 0-13-981176-1.

2. Dominguez de Villota ED, Ruiz Carmona MT, Rubio JJ, de Andrés S (December 1981). "Equality of the in vivo and in vitro oxygen-binding capacity of haemoglobin in patients with severe respiratory disease". *Br J Anaesth* **53** (12): 1325–8. PMID 7317251.

3. Costanzo, Linda S. (2007). *Physiology.* Hagerstwon, MD: Lippincott Williams & Wilkins. ISBN 0-7817-7311-3.

4. Hünefeld F.L. (1840). *Die Chemismus in der thierischen Organization.* Leipzig..

5. Funke O (1851). "Uber das milzvenenblut". *Z Rat Med* **1**: 172–218.

6. "A NASA Recipe For Protein Crystallography" (PDF). *Educational Brief.* National Aeronautics and Space Administration. http://www.okcareertech.org/cimc/special/nochild/downloads/science/Protein.Crystallography.pdf. Retrieved on 2008-10-12.

7. Hoppe-Seylor F (1866). "Uber die oxydation in lebendem blute". *Med-chem Untersuch Lab* **1**: 133–140.

8. Perutz, M.F.; Rossmann, M.G.; Cullis, A.F.; Muirhead, H.; Will, G.; North, A.C.T. (1960), "Structure of H", *Nature* **185** (4711): 416–422, doi:10.1038/185416a0

9. Perutz MF (November 1960). "Structure of hemoglobin". *Brookhaven symposia in biology* **13**: 165–83. PMID 13734651.

10. A Syllabus of Human Hemoglobin Variants (1996)

11. Hemoglobin Variants

12. Uthman, MD, Ed. "hemoglobinopathies and Thalassemias". http://web2.airmail.net/uthman/hemoglobinopathy/hemoglobinopathy.html. Retrieved on 2007-12-26.

13. "hemoglobin Synthesis". April 14, 2002. http://sickle.bwh.harvard.edu/hbsynthesis.html. Retrieved on 2007-12-26.

14. Steinberg 2001, p. 95

15. Hardison 1996, p. 1

16. Linberg R, Conover CD, Shum KL, Shorr RG (1998). "hemoglobin based oxygen carriers: how much methemoglobin is too much?". *Artif Cells Blood Substit Immobil Biotechnol* **26** (2): 133–48. PMID 9564432.

17. Van Beekvelt MC, Colier WN, Wevers RA, Van Engelen BG (2001). "Performance of near-infrared spectroscopy in measuring local O2 consumption and blood flow in skeletal muscle". *J Appl Physiol* **90** (2): 511–519. PMID 11160049.

18. Baillie/Simpson. "Online model of the haemoglobin binding and the effects of hyperventilation". http://www.altitude.org/calculators/saturationgraph/ saturationgraph.htm. Retrieved on 2006-08-10.

19. Childs PE (2001). "Haemoglobin - a molecular lung: 2". *Chemistry in Action* (65). ISSN 0332-2637. http://www.ul.ie/~childsp/CinA/Issue65/TOC28_ Haemoglobin.htm.

20. Guyton A C: Medical Physiology 11ed. 2005, page 509

21. Guyton, Arthur C.; John E. Hall (2006). *Textbook of Medical Physiology* (11 ed.). Philadelphia: Elsevier Saunders. p. 511. ISBN 0721602401.

22. Rang, H.P.; Dale M.M., Ritter J.M., Moore P.K. (2003). *Pharmacology, Fifth Edition.* Elsevier. ISBN 0443072027.

23. "hemoglobin Variants". *Lab Tests Online.* American Association for Clinical Chemistry. 2007-11-10. http://www.labtestsonline.org/understanding/ analytes/hemoglobin_var/glance-3.html. Retrieved on 2008-10-12.

24. Huisman THJ (1996). "A Syllabus of Human Hemoglobin Variants". *Globin Gene Server.* Pennsylvania State University. http://globin.cse.psu.edu/html/ huisman/variants/. Retrieved on 2008-10-12.

25. Johnson RA, Lavesa M, Askari B, Abraham NG, Nasjletti A (February 1995). "A heme oxygenase product, presumably carbon monoxide, mediates a vasodepressor function in rats". *Hypertension* **25** (2): 166–9. PMID 7843765. http://hyper.ahajournals.org/cgi/content/abstract/25/2/166. Retrieved on 2008-10-12.

26. *hemoglobinopathy* at Dorland's Medical Dictionary

27. britannica.com --> blood disease, stating *hypoxemia (reduced oxygen tension in the blood).* Retrieved on May 25, 2009

28. Biology-Online.org --> Dictionary » H » Hypoxemia last modified 00:05, 29 December 2008

29. Page 430 -> Pathophysiology of acute respiratory failure in Trauma By William C. Wilson, Christopher M. Grande, David B. Hoyt Edition: illustrated Published by CRC Press, 2007 ISBN 082472920X, 9780824729202 1384 pages

30. Hazards of hypoxemia: How to protect your patient from low oxygen levels In Nursing , May 1996 by McGaffigan, Patricia A

31. Hemoglobin at Medline Plus

32. Hemoglobin Level Test

33. Murray S.S. & McKinney E.S.(2006). *Foundations of Maternal-Newborn Nursing.* (4th ed., p 919).Philadelphia: Saunders Elsevier

34. "Hematocrit (HCT) or Packed Cell Volume (PCV)". *DoctorsLounge.com.* http:// www.doctorslounge.com/hematology/labs/hematocrit.htm. Retrieved on 2007-12-26.

35. This Hb A1c level is only useful in individuals who have red blood cells (RBCs) with normal survivals (i.e., normal half-life). In individuals with abnormal RBCs, whether due to abnormal hemoglobin molecules (such as Hemoglobin S in Sickle Cell Anemia) or RBC membrane defects - or other problems, the RBC half-life is frequently shortened. In these individuals an alternative test called "fructosamine level" can be used. It measures the degree of glycation (glucose binding) to albumin, the most common blood protein, and reflects average blood glucose levels over the previous 18–21 days, which is the half-life of albumin molecules in the circulation.

36. Weber RE, Vinogradov SN (2001). "Nonvertebrate hemoglobins: functions and molecular adaptations". *Physiol. Rev.* **81** (2): 569–628. PMID 11274340.

37. Zal F, Lallier FH, Green BN, Vinogradov SN, Toulmond A (1996). "The multi-hemoglobin system of the hydrothermal vent tube worm Riftia pachyptila. II. Complete polypeptide chain composition investigated by maximum entropy analysis of mass spectra". *J. Biol. Chem.* **271** (15): 8875–81. PMID 8621529.

38. Minic Z, Hervé G (2004). "Biochemical and enzymological aspects of the symbiosis between the deep-sea tubeworm Riftia pachyptila and its bacterial endosymbiont". *Eur. J. Biochem.* **271** (15): 3093–102. doi:10.1111/j.1432-1033.2004.04248.x. PMID 15265029.

39. Boh, Larry (2001). *Pharmacy Practice Manual: A Guide to the Clinical Experience.* Lippincott Williams & Wilkins. ISBN 0781725410.

40. Holden, Constance (30 September 2005). "Blood and Steel" (pdf). *Science* **309:** 2160. doi:10.1126/science.309.5744.2160d. http://www.sciencemag.org/cgi/reprint/309/5744/2160d.pdf.

GNU FREE DOCUMENTATION LICENSE

0. PREAMBLE

The purpose of this License is to make a manual, textbook, or other functional and useful document "free" in the sense of freedom: to assure everyone the effective freedom to copy and redistribute it, with or without modifying it, either commercially or noncommercially. Secondarily, this License preserves for the author and publisher a way to get credit for their work, while not being considered responsible for modifications made by others.

This License is a kind of "copyleft", which means that derivative works of the document must themselves be free in the same sense. It complements the GNU General Public License, which is a copyleft license designed for free software.

We have designed this License in order to use it for manuals for free software, because free software needs free documentation: a free program should come with manuals providing the same freedoms that the software does. But this License is not limited to software manuals; it can be used for any textual work, regardless of subject matter or whether it is published as a printed book. We recommend this License principally for works whose purpose is instruction or reference.

1. APPLICABILITY AND DEFINITIONS

This License applies to any manual or other work, in any medium, that contains a notice placed by the copyright holder saying it can be distributed under the terms of this License. Such a notice grants a world-wide, royalty-free license, unlimited in duration, to use that work under the conditions stated herein. The "Document", herein, refers to any such manual or work. Any member of the public is a licensee, and is addressed as "you". You accept the license if you copy, modify or distribute the work in a way requiring permission under copyright law.

A "Modified Version" of the Document means any work containing the Document or a portion of it, either copied verbatim, or with modifications and/or translated into another language.

A "Secondary Section" is a named appendix or a front-matter section of the Document that deals exclusively with the relationship of the publishers or authors of the Document to the Document's overall subject (or to related matters) and contains nothing that could fall directly within that overall subject. (Thus, if the Document is in part a textbook of mathematics, a Secondary Section may not explain any mathematics.) The relationship could be a matter of historical connection with the subject or with related matters, or of legal, commercial, philosophical, ethical or political position regarding them.

The "Invariant Sections" are certain Secondary Sections whose titles are designated, as being those of Invariant Sections, in the notice that says that the Document is released under this License. If a section does not fit the above definition of Secondary then it is not allowed to be designated as Invariant. The Document may contain zero Invariant Sections. If the Document does not identify any Invariant Sections then there are none.

The "Cover Texts" are certain short passages of text that are listed, as Front-Cover Texts or Back-Cover Texts, in the notice that says that the Document is released under this License. A Front-Cover Text may be at most 5 words, and a Back-Cover Text may be at most 25 words.

A "Transparent" copy of the Document means a machine-readable copy, represented in a format whose specification is available to the general public, that is suitable for revising the document straightforwardly with generic text editors or (for images composed of pixels) generic paint programs or (for drawings) some widely available drawing editor, and that is suitable for input to text formatters or for automatic translation to a variety of formats suitable for input to text formatters. A copy made in an otherwise Transparent file format whose markup, or absence of markup, has been arranged to thwart or discourage subsequent modification by readers is not Transparent. An image format is not Transparent if used for any substantial amount of text. A copy that is not "Transparent" is called "Opaque".

Examples of suitable formats for Transparent copies include plain ASCII without markup, Texinfo input format, LaTeX input format, SGML or XML using a publicly available DTD, and standard-conforming simple HTML, PostScript or PDF designed for human modification. Examples of transparent image formats include PNG, XCF and JPG. Opaque formats include proprietary formats that can be read and edited only by proprietary word processors, SGML or XML for which the DTD and/or processing tools are not generally available, and the machine-generated HTML, PostScript or PDF produced by some word processors for output purposes only.

The "Title Page" means, for a printed book, the title page itself, plus such following pages as are needed to hold, legibly, the material this License requires to appear in the title page. For works in formats which do not have any title page as such, "Title Page" means the text near the most prominent appearance of the work's title, preceding the beginning of the body of the text.

A section "Entitled XYZ" means a named subunit of the Document whose title either is precisely XYZ or contains XYZ in parentheses following text that translates XYZ in another language. (Here XYZ stands for a specific section name mentioned below, such as "Acknowledgements", "Dedications", "Endorsements", or "History".) To "Preserve the Title" of such a section when you modify the Document means that it remains a section "Entitled XYZ" according to this definition.

The Document may include Warranty Disclaimers next to the notice which states that this License applies to the Document. These Warranty Disclaimers are considered to be included by reference in this License, but only as regards disclaiming warranties: any other implication that these Warranty Disclaimers may have is void and has no effect on the meaning of this License.

2. VERBATIM COPYING

You may copy and distribute the Document in any medium, either commercially or noncommercially, provided that this License, the copyright notices, and the license notice saying this License applies to the Document are reproduced in all copies, and that you add no other conditions whatsoever to those of this License. You may not use technical measures to obstruct or control the reading or further copying of the copies you make or distribute. However, you may accept compensation in exchange for copies. If you distribute a large enough number of copies you must also follow the conditions in section 3.

You may also lend copies, under the same conditions stated above, and you may publicly display copies.

3. COPYING IN QUANTITY

If you publish printed copies (or copies in media that commonly have printed covers) of the Document, numbering more than 100, and the Document's license notice requires Cover Texts, you must enclose the copies in covers that carry, clearly and legibly, all these Cover Texts: Front-Cover Texts on the front cover, and Back-Cover Texts on the back cover. Both covers must also clearly and legibly identify you as the publisher of these copies. The front cover must present the full title with all words of the title equally prominent and visible. You may add other material on the covers in addition. Copying with changes limited to the covers, as long as they preserve the title of the Document and satisfy these conditions, can be treated as verbatim copying in other respects.

If the required texts for either cover are too voluminous to fit legibly, you should put the first ones listed (as many as fit reasonably) on the actual cover, and continue the rest onto adjacent pages.

If you publish or distribute Opaque copies of the Document numbering more than 100, you must either include a machine-readable Transparent copy along with each Opaque copy, or state in or with each Opaque copy a computer-network location from which the general network-using public has access to download using public-standard network protocols a complete Transparent copy of the Document, free of added material. If you use the latter option, you must take reasonably prudent steps, when you begin distribution of Opaque copies in quantity, to ensure that this Transparent copy will remain thus accessible at the stated location until at least one year after the last time you distribute an Opaque copy (directly or through your agents or retailers) of that edition to the public.

It is requested, but not required, that you contact the authors of the Document well before redistributing any large number of copies, to give them a chance to provide you with an updated version of the Document.

4. MODIFICATIONS

You may copy and distribute a Modified Version of the Document under the conditions of sections 2 and 3 above, provided that you release the Modified Version under precisely this License, with the Modified Version filling the role of the Document, thus licensing distribution and modification of the Modified Version to whoever possesses a copy of it. In addition, you must do these things in the Modified Version:

A. Use in the Title Page (and on the covers, if any) a title distinct from that of the Document, and from those of previous versions (which should, if there were any, be listed in the History section of the Document). You may use the same title as a previous version if the original publisher of that version gives permission.

B. List on the Title Page, as authors, one or more persons or entities responsible for authorship of the modifications in the Modified Version, together with at least five of the principal authors of the Document (all of its principal authors, if it has fewer than five), unless they release you from this requirement.

C. State on the Title page the name of the publisher of the Modified Version, as the publisher.

D. Preserve all the copyright notices of the Document.

E. Add an appropriate copyright notice for your modifications adjacent to the other copyright notices.

F. Include, immediately after the copyright notices, a license notice giving the public permission to use the Modified Version under the terms of this License, in the form shown in the Addendum below.

G. Preserve in that license notice the full lists of Invariant Sections and required Cover Texts given in the Document's license notice.

H. Include an unaltered copy of this License.

I. Preserve the section Entitled "History", Preserve its Title, and add to it an item stating at least the title, year, new authors, and publisher of the Modified Version as given on the Title Page. If there is no section Entitled "History" in the Document, create one stating the title, year, authors, and publisher of the Document as given on its Title Page, then add an item describing the Modified Version as stated in the previous sentence.

J. Preserve the network location, if any, given in the Document for public access to a Transparent copy of the Document, and likewise the network locations given in the Document for previous versions it was based on. These may be placed in the "History" section. You may omit a network location for a work that was published at least four years before the Document itself, or if the original publisher of the version it refers to gives permission.

K. For any section entitled "Acknowledgements" or "Dedications", Preserve the Title of the section, and preserve in the section all the substance and tone of each of the contributor acknowledgements and/or dedications given therein.

L. Preserve all the Invariant Sections of the Document, unaltered in their text and in their titles. Section numbers or the equivalent are not considered part of the section titles.

M. Delete any section entitled "Endorsements". Such a section may not be included in the Modified Version.

N. Do not retitle any existing section to be entitled "Endorsements" or to conflict in title with any Invariant Section.

O. Preserve any Warranty Disclaimers.

If the Modified Version includes new front-matter sections or appendices that qualify as Secondary Sections and contain no material copied from the Document, you may at your option designate some or all of these sections as Invariant. To do this, add their titles to the list of Invariant Sections in the Modified Version's license notice. These titles must be distinct from any other section titles.

You may add a section entitled "Endorsements", provided it contains nothing but endorsements of your Modified Version by various parties—for example, statements of peer review or that the text has been approved by an organization as the authoritative definition of a standard.

You may add a passage of up to five words as a Front-Cover Text, and a passage of up to 25 words as a Back-Cover Text, to the end of the list of Cover Texts in the Modified Version. Only one passage of Front-Cover Text and one of Back-Cover Text may be added by (or through arrangements made by) any one entity. If the Document already includes a Cover Text for the same cover, previously added by you or by arrangement made by the same entity you are acting on behalf of, you may not add another; but you may replace the old one, on explicit permission from the previous publisher that added the old one.

The author(s) and publisher(s) of the Document do not by this License give permission to use their names for publicity for or to assert or imply endorsement of any Modified Version.

5. COMBINING DOCUMENTS

You may combine the Document with other documents released under this License, under the terms defined in section 4 above for modified versions, provided that you include in the combination all of the Invariant Sections of all of the original documents, unmodified, and list them all as Invariant Sections of your combined work in its license notice, and that you preserve all their Warranty Disclaimers.

The combined work need only contain one copy of this License, and multiple identical Invariant Sections may be replaced with a single copy. If there are multiple Invariant Sections with the same name but different contents, make the title of each such section unique by adding at the end of it, in parentheses, the name of the original author or publisher of that section if known, or else a unique number. Make the same adjustment to the section titles in the list of Invariant Sections in the license notice of the combined work.

In the combination, you must combine any sections entitled "History" in the various original documents, forming one section entitled "History";

likewise combine any sections entitled "Acknowledgements", and any sections entitled "Dedications". You must delete all sections entitled "Endorsements."

6. COLLECTIONS OF DOCUMENTS

You may make a collection consisting of the Document and other documents released under this License, and replace the individual copies of this License in the various documents with a single copy that is included in the collection, provided that you follow the rules of this License for verbatim copying of each of the documents in all other respects.

You may extract a single document from such a collection, and distribute it individually under this License, provided you insert a copy of this License into the extracted document, and follow this License in all other respects regarding verbatim copying of that document.

7. AGGREGATION WITH INDEPENDENT WORKS

A compilation of the Document or its derivatives with other separate and independent documents or works, in or on a volume of a storage or distribution medium, is called an "aggregate" if the copyright resulting from the compilation is not used to limit the legal rights of the compilation's users beyond what the individual works permit. When the Document is included in an aggregate, this License does not apply to the other works in the aggregate which are not themselves derivative works of the Document.

If the Cover Text requirement of section 3 is applicable to these copies of the Document, then if the Document is less than one half of the entire aggregate, the Document's Cover Texts may be placed on covers that bracket the Document within the aggregate, or the electronic equivalent of covers if the Document is in electronic form. Otherwise they must appear on printed covers that bracket the whole aggregate.

8. TRANSLATION

Translation is considered a kind of modification, so you may distribute translations of the Document under the terms of section 4. Replacing Invariant Sections with translations requires special permission from their copyright holders, but you may include translations of some or all Invariant Sections in addition to the original versions of these Invariant Sections. You may include a translation of this License, and all the license notices in the Document, and any Warranty Disclaimers, provided that you also include the original English version of this License and the original versions of those notices and disclaimers. In case of a disagreement between the translation and the original version of this License or a notice or disclaimer, the original version will prevail.

If a section in the Document is entitled "Acknowledgements", "Dedications", or "History", the requirement (section 4) to Preserve its Title (section 1) will typically require changing the actual title.

9. TERMINATION

You may not copy, modify, sublicense, or distribute the Document except as expressly provided for under this License. Any other attempt to copy, modify, sublicense or distribute the Document is void, and will automatically terminate your rights under this License. However, parties who have received copies, or rights, from you under this License will not have their licenses terminated so long as such parties remain in full compliance.

10. FUTURE REVISIONS OF THIS LICENSE

The Free Software Foundation may publish new, revised versions of the GNU Free Documentation License from time to time. Such new versions will be similar in spirit to the present version, but may differ in detail to address new problems or concerns. See http://www.gnu.org/copyleft/.

Each version of the License is given a distinguishing version number. If the Document specifies that a particular numbered version of this License "or any later version" applies to it, you have the option of following the terms and conditions either of that specified version or of any later version that has been published (not as a draft) by the Free Software Foundation. If the Document does not specify a version number of this License, you may choose any version ever published (not as a draft) by the Free Software Foundation.

INDEX

www.ingramcontent.com/pod-product-compliance
Lightning Source LLC
Chambersburg PA
CBHW070806290326
41931CB00011BA/2153